Heaven's Lifestyle Today

Health in the Context of Revelation 14

A Biblical and Modern Science Perspective

P. William Dysinger, M.D., M.P.H.

The Ministerial Association
General Conference of Seventh-day Adventists
Silver Spring, MD 20904

CONTENTS

FOREWORD

More than forty years ago I graduated from the College of Medical Evangelists in Loma Linda, California, and began a medical ministry which has taken me to more than 120 countries around the world. My interest and experiences have focused especially on the poorest countries of the earth. I have been profoundly impressed that God's plan of health is simple and appropriate to all people everywhere.

For years I have taken a special interest in the relationship between health and the three angels' messages in Revelation 14. Ellen G. White frequently emphasized this relationship:

> The health reform, I was shown, is a part of the **third angel's message** and is just as closely connected with it as are the arm and hand with the human body. I saw that we as a people must make an advance move in this great work. Ministers and people must act in concert. God's people are not prepared for the loud cry of the **third angel**. They have a work to do for themselves which they should not leave for God to do for them. He has left the work for them to do.
>
> *Testimonies for the Church,* vol. 1, p. 486

> To make natural law plain, and to urge obedience to it, is a work that accompanies the **third angel's message**. . . . He designs that the subject shall be agitated and the public mind deeply stirred to investigate it. . . . He who cherishes the light which God has given him upon health reform has an important aid in the work of becoming sanctified through the truth and fitted for immortality.
>
> *Counsels on Health,* pp. 21, 22

> I was again shown that the health reform is one branch of the great work which is to fit a people for the coming of the Lord. It is as closely connected with the **third angel's message** as the hand is with the body. . . . Men and women cannot violate natural law by indulging depraved appetite and lustful passions, and not violate the law of God. . . . To make plain natural law, and urge the obedience of it, is the work that accompanies the **third angel's message** to prepare a people for the coming of the Lord.
>
> *Testimonies for the Church,* vol. 3, p. 161

Combine medical missionary work with the proclamation of the **third angel's message**. Make regular, organized efforts to lift the church members out of the dead level in which they have been for years. Send out into the churches workers who will live the principles of health reform. Let those be sent who can see the necessity of self-denial in appetite, or they will be a snare to the church. See if the breath of life will not then come into our churches.

Testimonies for the Church, vol. 6, p. 267

As we near **the close of time**, we must rise higher and still higher upon the question of health reform and Christian temperance, presenting it in a more positive and decided manner. We must strive continually to educate the people, not only by our words but by our practice.

Testimonies for the Church, vol. 6, p. 112

These and other similar statements show the important relationship between health work and the messages of the angels in Revelation 14. Only recently, however, has God impressed me that the three angels' messages present a framework for teaching basic health principles for body and mind.

This framework is not meant in any way to be a comprehensive exposition of the three angels' messages. I have purposely refrained from getting into a discussion of the "beast and his image" and other doctrinal topics not pertinent to health. I simply give a literal health interpretation to each phrase in the messages of the three angels.

This framework provides an atmosphere of powerful motivation to health education. Facts and philosophy are freely mixed. Great importance is placed on learning to live a sanctified lifestyle here on earth, in preparation for heaven. Also emphasized is the fact that character—the only trait taken directly from earth to heaven—is mostly developed by the small decisions of routine, daily living.

Although presented in a Biblical framework, modern health science findings are presented in this book. There should be no embarrassment in discussing these with educated health scientists. While an attempt is made to be as detailed as possible, the book's size limitations prevent going very far beyond basic health principles.

The inspired writings of Ellen G. White are quoted only occasionally. However, I hope this Biblical study will encourage deep exploration of the marvelous insights into health that God gave this modern prophet. This book supplements and complements health books such as *The Ministry of Healing*.

It is my desire that this book will instill in each reader awe and respect for God's creation in human bodies. I hope that readers will make a commitment to glorify God by a healthy lifestyle. The book is also intended as a reliable reference text for practical sermons and seminars.

I pray that God's way will be clearly seen in our lives and that His name will be glorified on earth in preparation for His soon coming.

P. William Dysinger, M.D., M.P.H.
684 Dry Prong Road
Williamsport, TN 38487

CREDITS

I was very fortunate to obtain the reviewers I sought. These included Jeris M. Bragan, an accomplished author I much admire; Norman Gulley, Ph.D., an eschatologist in whom I have much faith; Mervyn G. Hardinge, M.D., Dr.P.H., Ph.D., my long-term mentor during the years I was his associate at the School of Public Health, Loma Linda, California; William Shea, M.D., Ph.D., a member of the Biblical Research Institute and both a physician and a theologian; Mike Speegle, an associate in the Ministerial Association of the General Conference of Seventh-day Adventists; and Albert S. Whiting, M.D., M.P.H., director of the Health and Temperance Department of the General Conference of Seventh-day Adventists. You have all given me valuable counsel and insights and have provided me feedback I greatly appreciate. Many thanks for your assistance and encouragement!

DEDICATION

My life and study have been profoundly influenced by my family, and I love you all. This book is especially dedicated to you, Edwin, Wayne, and John. You have been much in my thoughts during the study for this book. Your dedication to God and His service, your desire to prepare for Christ's soon coming, and your commitment to raise your children in the nurture and admonition of the Lord have been particularly inspiring. May this book be a special blessing to you and your families. May you sense something of the excitement and deep feelings that were mine as God's Spirit opened new thoughts to me from His written Word and His book of nature. Thank you for all you mean to me. Accept this little book as a token of my love for each of you.

CHAPTER ONE

The Gospel to Every People

THEN I SAW ANOTHER ANGEL FLYING IN THE MIDST OF HEAVEN, HAVING THE EVER-LASTING GOSPEL TO PREACH TO THOSE WHO DWELL ON THE EARTH—TO EVERY NATION, TRIBE, TONGUE, AND PEOPLE. REVELATION 14:6.

Revelation 14 sends a special message to people living on earth at the end of time. The chapter begins by describing the 144,000—those who were "redeemed from among men, being firstfruits to God and to the Lamb"[1]— and ends by portraying Christ's second coming. In the middle lies the message of three angels flying in the "midst of heaven, having the everlasting gospel to preach to those who dwell on the earth—to every nation, tribe, tongue and people."[2] The angels speak "with a loud voice,"[3] indicating that this message is meant for every person on earth in the last days.

This book is not intended to provide a comprehensive theology of these messages. Instead, our discussion focuses on health implications. Within this area we find a deep and vital message for God's people today. Because the ultimate purpose in health education is "to prepare a people for the coming of the Lord,"[4] the messages of the three angels form an ideal framework for teaching health. Health presented in this context combines basic principles with a powerful motivation to live one's religion. The result is a practical, vivid description of sanctified living.

In His Image

The everlasting gospel (good news) begins with the knowledge that we are created by God in His image.[5] A loving God chose to create beings who could love and appreciate Him, even as He loved them. He wanted them to be His friends, to walk and talk with Him in the beautiful garden He had made.

Since a love relationship cannot be forced, God accepted the risk of creating individuals who could not only procreate themselves physically but could also create new thoughts and actions. Humans were designed to choose for themselves how best to love God and how to show that love in word and action.

God foresaw that man alone was not sufficiently representative of Him. He said, "It is not good that man should be alone."[6] It takes the unique characteristics of both male and female to be like Him.[7] How beautifully man and woman complement each other. Their strength is in their ability to truly become one in spirit, to think and work together as one.

God created humans in His likeness, with the ability to grow and develop every capability—physical, mental, and spiritual. The intended purpose of life is to glorify God by living to bless others.

The Fall

Lucifer originated selfishness in heaven itself and recruited a third of the angels to his side. Like Lucifer, they doubted God and rejected His goodness. Satan (the fallen Lucifer) successfully convinced the angels to view God as severe and unforgiving. Then he turned his attention to God's newly created beings on earth.

God allowed humans to choose whether to obey or to accept temptation. In effect God said, "If you love Me, you will want to do what I ask and avoid what is harmful." Temptation was restricted to one tree in the midst of the garden. Adam and Eve were warned, "but of the tree of knowledge of good and evil you shall not eat, for in the day that you eat of it you shall surely die."[8] God, in His love, sought to discourage their contact with Satan. His laws are given for our protection. They are not arbitrary dictums, but reminders of His loving care.

Sin entered earth when Eve, enjoying the beautiful garden, wandered away from Adam and found herself alone by the forbidden tree. Satan's appearance as a beautiful talking serpent caught her attention. (Incidentally, there is reason to believe the original serpents were much more like beautiful birds than the groveling snakes we know today.) The cunning devil began appealing to her human curiosity—her desire to gain knowledge. Knowing this desire, the serpent urged her to judge for herself what "was good for food and . . . pleasant to the eyes, and . . . desirable to make one wise."[9] The record says, Eve "took of its fruit and ate. She also gave to her husband with her, and he ate."[10]

Satan boldly encouraged doubt of God's truthfulness. People naturally seek their own desires above that which is for the common good or that which is dictated by divine revelation. We all seek to be our own gods, deciding for ourselves what is good and what is evil. The devil convinces us that if it "looks good, tastes good, and feels good," it must be good. For six thousand years since Eden, personal desire, appetite, and passion have ruled human hearts—and we die prematurely as a result. However, God has prepared a way of escape.

Good News

God did not make humans in His image and then abandon them when they sinned. The good news is that Jesus chose to take our sentence so that all who accept Him can live eternally. Because Satan's misrepresentation of God as severe and unforgiving could not be easily overcome, God sent His Son, the only One who fully knew and could fully reveal the height and depth of divine love for humans. Sin had marred and almost obliterated the image of God in humans. It was to restore this image that the plan of salvation was devised. The return of humans to the perfection in which they were created is the great object of life in Christ.[11]

There is more good news. God has made a "way of escape" from the temptations which so frequently beset us.[12] We find an example in the life of Jesus, who overcame at every point in which Adam and Eve and their descendants failed. The devil particularly tempted our Lord in the wilderness as He fasted and prayed before beginning His public ministry. Significantly, the temptations were in the areas of appetite and human desire, the very areas in which Adam and Eve failed. These remain our most common areas of sin, and the three angels give their messages to help us overcome these temptations.

The ultimate good news is that Jesus not only set an example but wants to directly assist us. Christ in us (through His spirit) is our only "hope of glory."[13] Only with His help can we live a holy life. His graphically expresses His desire for us in His prayer in John 17: "I in them, and You in Me; that they may be perfect. . . ."[14] Paul indicates that this perfection is one of body, as well as spirit, and that Christ overcomes for us. "Now may the God of peace Himself *sanctify you completely*; and may your whole spirit, soul, *and body* be preserved blameless at the coming of our Lord Jesus Christ. He who calls you is faithful, *who also will do it*."[15]

Renewal and Restoration

God wants not only for us to overcome, but also to restore us to the image in which we were created. Christian health workers should never be satisfied with simply helping sick people overcome pain or recover their previous level of health. The goal is to help everyone reach ever higher levels of health, to take steps toward increased development of body, mind, and soul—toward the restoration of God's image in humans. This obviously requires more than treating symptoms. It requires us to identify the cause of illness and help people make lifestyle changes that can repair damage, prevent disease, and promote health.

This approach to health holds great spiritual significance. We learn to better understand God and our relationship with Him. The study of our bodies teaches us that God expects a balance between the two beliefs that we can (a) know and fully obey the laws of nature and thus earn health by our own efforts versus the other extreme in which (b) we expect a miraculous healing simply because God loves us and will heal regardless of our chosen lifestyle.

In these last days our work for God includes teaching people to understand the principles of health. We must show that following Satan's way and disobeying God's laws, physical or moral, leads to disease and death, while following God's way leads to life and health. By and large, it is in the many small choices of daily living that we develop character and prepare for eternity. Sanctification is not just a theory. It's living day by day, minute by minute, in such a way that we know we are following God's will in everything. This isn't easy, and Paul describes it thus: "I discipline my body and bring it into subjection, lest, when I have preached to others, I myself should become disqualified."[16] But praise God, we don't have to do it on our own. "I can do all things through Christ who strengthens me."[17]

David makes clear that God doesn't distinguish between disease of body and sin of soul. In one breath, both forgiveness and healing are proclaimed: "Bless the Lord . . . who forgives all your iniquities, who heals all your diseases, who redeems your life from destruction." He is the God "who satisfies your mouth with good things, so that your youth is renewed like the eagle's."[18] Isaiah says those who wait on God will "renew their strength."[19] Restoration is our goal! In fact, Peter points out that the "restoration of all things" has been the theme of all the prophets.[20]

The everlasting gospel of the first angel includes the proclamation that God made us in His image, and even though we have tarnished that image by our poor lifestyles, He plans to restore us if we will cooperate with Him.

Fearfully and Wonderfully Made

Despite the degeneration that began in Eden, many years later the Psalmist was still able to proclaim,

> I praise You because I am fearfully and wonderfully made; your works are wonderful, I know that full well. My frame was not hidden from you when I was made in the secret place. When I was woven together in the depths of the earth, your eyes saw my unformed body. All the days ordained for me were written in your book before one of them came to be.[21]

Even today, three thousand years later, God can be known through His creation. Paul points out that "the invisible things of Him from the creation of the world are clearly seen, being understood by the things that are made, even His eternal power and Godhead; so that they are without excuse. . . ."[22]

We would do well to study God's creation, the human body, to learn of His greatness. A study of anatomy and physiology helps clarify the plan of salvation, especially the delicate mix between God's grace and our works. Through nature we learn that human life is controlled by the laws of nature. God is as much the author of natural, physical laws as He is the author of moral laws. The need to understand the sanctity of God's physical laws becomes ever more crucial as we near the end of the world.

Thread of Life

Deoxyribonucleic acid (DNA) reveals the remarkable wisdom of the Creator. David describes DNA well when he says, "My frame was not hidden from you when I was made in the secret place. . . . Your eyes saw my unformed body. All the days ordained for me were written in your book before one of them came to be."[23]

Often called the "thread of life," DNA is an amazing chemical molecule residing in the nucleus of each of our trillions of body cells. Although comparatively simple, it contains the code of everything a person inherits and is a manual of all body structures and functions. It consists of a ladderlike chemical substance, in which the sides of the ladder are made up of alternating molecules of phosphoric acid (P) and the sugar, deoxyribose (D). The rungs between the strands are made up of four protein bases: adenine (A), thiamine (T), guanine (G), and cytosine (C). In these rungs, A is always loosely attached to T, and G to C.

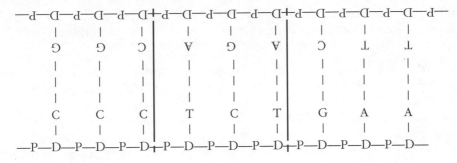

Figure 1. *Small portion of DNA molecule. (See text for code.)*

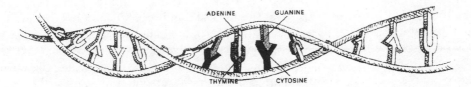

Figure 2. *Helical (coiled) shape of DNA. (To put DNA in its proper physical perspective, one merely needs to pick up the two ends and twist them into a helix. Ten pairs of nucleotides are present in each full turn of the helix.)*

A nucleotide is a combination of one molecule of phosphoric acid and a molecule of deoxyribose with one of the four bases—A, T, G, or C. The many combinations of these four bases make up "the code of life." Thousands of these rungs or "steps" make a gene. Each DNA molecule contains about 200,000 different genes (or gene slots).

Some six billion "steps" of DNA in a single cell record each person's anatomic and physiologic blueprint. Although arranged in spiral form, each DNA molecule would be six feet long if stretched out, but it is tightly packed to fit and function in the nucleolus, a space measuring 1/2,500 of an inch (1/1,000 of a centimeter). It doesn't just lie there, however. It bends and twists a billion times a second while its ladder sides "breathe" in and out.[24] This dramatic dance allows RNA (ribonucleic acid) particles to make contact with the portion of the DNA molecule that gives them their up-to-date instructions for making the protein/enzymes which direct cell functions. (DNA can be compared to an architect whose job is to draw up and manage the grand design. RNA is the contractor who takes orders from the architect and communicates with all parts of the cell.)

Each person's DNA is the same in every cell of his or her body. For instance, the DNA in a skin cell is the same as the DNA in a nerve cell or a muscle cell. Each cell contains all the information needed to reproduce a complete human being.

A mystery we are only beginning to understand relates to cell development after conception. How that first cell (and the small cluster of non-specialized cells that develops in the first few days after the ovum is fertilized) multiplies into the trillions of specialized cells that make up a complex human is truly miraculous. At some point in early fetal development, the DNA in each cell decides that one cell will begin to make a heart, another will begin to make a finger, and another, a nerve cell. Each person on earth is different from every other because each has a unique DNA molecule with its own schedule of development.

DNA controls both the reproduction and the day-by-day function of all cells. Each adult body contains up to 100 trillion cells, millions of which die every second and must be replaced. For instance, cells making up the lining of the intestines live only a day and a half, white blood cells live about 13 days, and red blood cells live up to 120 days. The only exception to this death and reproduction cycle is in the nervous system, where nerve cells, if they die or are killed, are not replaced. DNA also controls the manufacturing of enzymes or chemicals which give each cell its specific characteristics—sensation of light in the eye, taste on the tongue, digestive juices in the intestine, detoxification in the liver, movement in muscles, and so on.

Consider for a moment what functions are included in each DNA molecule. The instructions in one DNA molecule, if spelled out in words, would fill several sets of encyclopedias. Despite this enormous amount of information, the physical amount of DNA is small. Some estimate that the DNA of all five billion people alive today could fit into a teaspoon weighing only one twenty-fifth of an ounce.[25]

We will consider three categories of functions: (a) growth and development; (b) unique characteristics; and (c) cellular activities.

Growth and development. From the moment of conception, when the male sperm unites with the female ovum, the resulting DNA molecule determines the speed and time of each cell division. At first each new cell looks identical, but at a time determined by the DNA, cells begin to differentiate and reproduce at different rates. By the third week after conception, most of the 600 types of specialized cells have begun differentiating themselves from each other. By week four, the brain can begin to be recognized, the heart and intestinal tract are being formed, the arm and leg stumps are visible, and the kidneys appear. The head is almost half the total length of the body by week five, and the two hemispheres of the brain are easily seen. The heart begins pumping. By week six, nerve connections are linking up at the rate of 250,000 per minute, the eyes and ears are well-formed, the mouth has taken shape, and the skeleton begins to form. By week seven, the teeth buds are visible, the stomach begins secreting digestive acid, and the fingers and toes are differentiated. And by the end of the eighth week, differentiation into specialized cells is essentially complete. The remaining seven months is spent mostly in growing, not developing new tissues.

Not only is fetal development scheduled in DNA, but the life pattern is also there. When the child will be born and how soon it can be expected to turn over in bed, crawl, walk, and talk are all programmed in DNA. When puberty will occur, how soon men will begin to grow facial hair (or lose the hair on top), when gray hair will appear, and the expected length of life are also programmed. Environment can influence some of these developments, but each person is programmed with an individual schedule inherited from parents.

Unique characteristics. Each individual's DNA encodes the family and racial characteristics handed down for generations. These include skin color, height, nose shape, eye and hair color, weight tendencies, and a multitude of other characteristics. Increasingly we see that many behavior patterns are also inherited, including personality types and the way we laugh or walk. Some people inherit tendencies toward heart disease, diabetes, or other chronic disease. There are about 1,800 genetically determined diseases, such as sickle-cell disease, thalassemia, and Down's syndrome.

Cellular activities. The cell is the basic element of life. All bodily function is determined by a person's cells and the enzymes that control their functions. Which substances will be synthesized within each cell is determined by DNA. As we think of the body's numerous activities—the hormonal functions of the glandular cells, the detoxifying ability of liver and kidney cells, the movement function of muscle cells, and so on—we see that they are all dependent on the programming ability of DNA. Although each cell holds instructions for every cell in the body, it somehow uses only the portion of DNA code needed for its own individual function.

DNA also monitors cell walls to ensure that only the needed nutrients pass through. And it maintains a balance between all functions. The heart does not beat faster or harder than needed for the current level of activity. A certain level of thyroid is maintained in the blood. Different types of saliva are produced as different kinds of food are ingested. Male and female hormones are produced in proper amounts. Blood sugar levels are maintained.

All of this is programmed by DNA. Although essential to life, it can be affected by lifestyle and environment. For instance, radiation and toxic chemicals can damage DNA and alter the code of life, causing some cells to begin the wild growth we recognize as cancer. Some viruses are actually foreign counterfeit DNA or RNA particles which enter cells and cause DNA to send wrong signals and alter functions.

It is good news to know how fearfully and wonderfully we are made. The good news of the three angels' messages includes the knowledge that the God who encoded our DNA is worthy of trust and devotion. We show our love and gratitude by caring for the amazing bodies He gave us.

---

[1] Revelation 14:4.
[2] Revelation 14:6.
[3] Revelation 14:7.
[4] Ellen G. White, *Testimonies for the Church,* vol. 3 (Pacific Press, 1948) 161.
[5] Genesis 1:27.
[6] Genesis 2:18.
[7] Genesis 1:27.
[8] Genesis 2:17.
[9] Genesis 3:6.
[10] Ibid.
[11] Ellen G. White, *Education* (Pacific Press, 1903) 15, 16.
[12] 1 Corinthians 10:13.
[13] Colossians 1:27.
[14] John 17:23.
[15] 1 Thessalonians 5:23, 24.
[16] 1 Corinthians 9:27.
[17] Philippians 4:13.
[18] Psalm 103:1-5.
[19] Isaiah 40:31.
[20] Acts 3:21.
[21] Psalm 139:14-16 (NIV).
[22] Romans 1:20.
[23] Psalm 139:16.
[24] "Beginning the Journey," *The Incredible Machine* (National Geographic Society, 1986) 43.
[25] David Bodanis, *The Body Book: A Fantastic Voyage to the World Within* (Little, Brown & Co., 1984) 115.

CHAPTER TWO

Fear God

SAYING WITH A LOUD VOICE, "FEAR GOD. . . ." REVELATION 14:7 (FIRST PART).

The first words of the first angel of Revelation 14 are "Fear God."[1] God obviously feels it important that we humans approach Him with awe and reverence. The Psalmist says, "The fear of the Lord is the beginning of wisdom."[2] This recommended fear does not include anxiety, dismay, dread, or terror. Only the devil views a loving God in such ways. While the devil tries to portray God as vengeful and severe, God identifies Himself as "The Lord, the Lord God, merciful and gracious, long-suffering, and abounding in goodness and truth."[3]

Recognizing God as Creator leads us to seek knowledge of Him through what He has made. The human body, the wonder of creation, is a logical place to begin our study. Seeking to learn of God makes the study of anatomy and physiology very meaningful. The work of a master engineer becomes evident, showing that our bodies could not have evolved simply through chance or random evolution. DNA is a good illustration of God's awesome power. Here are two others:

The Eye

Perhaps the best example demonstrating the difficulty of belief in random evolution is the eye. The eye is a wonderful organ, but only if it is all there. It could not have developed from single small changes because many changes would have been needed simultaneously, both to the eye and surrounding structures.[4]

Except in rare instances genetic changes cause reduction, loss, or impairment of body structures, processes, and viability. Beneficial natural selection could only operate in those exceedingly rare instances where a change confers an advantage. . . . Progressive evolution must show a long series of small intermediate changes. . . . For the origin of delicately balanced interrelated systems (such as the eye and vision), this poses a well-nigh insurmountable obstacle.[5]

Marvelous design is seen in the eye. Light travels through the pupil to the retina in the back of the eye. There it is registered chemically in the rod and cone cells, which transmit sight through nerves to the back of the skull where we "see" in the posterior (occipital) lobe of the brain. The ability to see is tremendously complex, so we will illustrate by describing just the muscular actions necessary for vision.

The eyes are never truly still. If an image was held stationary on the retina, the participating photoreceptors (rods and cones) would soon be chemically fatigued, and the image would fade. Continuous, small, rapid eye movements guarantee that an image constantly sweeps across the retina to be processed by fresh photoreceptors. The exterior (extrinsic) eye muscles make these movements possible.

Each eye is equipped with three pairs of taut, elastic muscles. As with other skeletal muscles of the body, which almost all work in pairs, each eye muscle vies with its counterpart to pull the eye in different directions. The superior rectus diverts the gaze upward, while the inferior rectus pulls downward. The lateral rectus swivels the eye outward, while the medial rectus swivels toward the nose. The superior and inferior oblique muscles roll the eyes clockwise or counter-clockwise. Among them, these six muscles allow eye movement in every direction.

Each eye muscle originates on bone within the eye socket and attaches to the eyeball itself, just behind the pupil. Constant tension helps make these eye muscles among the fastest in the body. Capable of seven coordinated movements, they give humans one of nature's most advanced tracking systems. These muscles enable us to maintain binocular vision—the ability to visualize depth and distance.

An important eye muscle is the superior oblique muscle, which can only function by virtue of the muscle having a tendon which passes through a pulley-like growth of bone. This allows the muscle to be active at an almost 90-degree angle. (See Figure 3.) It is inconceivable that this muscle could have evolved an ability to grow and work through a bone pulley by accident. It is one of the myriad examples that support belief in a Creator God.

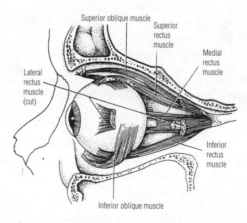

Figure 3. *The extrinsic muscles of the eye. Note the "pulley" used by the superior oblique muscle.*

Red Blood Cells

One of the simplest of all body cells is the red blood cell (RBC). RBCs are the most important single constituent of blood. Some 25 trillion of these tiny cells course through our 60,000 miles of blood vessels and make up about 45 percent of the blood's volume of six quarts. RBCs consist primarily of water and hemoglobin; the latter enables blood to carry oxygen efficiently from the lungs to each body cell and to return carbon dioxide from cells to lungs. RBCs are produced in the red bone marrow and live about four months (120 days), during which time each RBC travels between lungs and body tissues 75,000 times before returning to the bone marrow to die.[6] About 3 million RBCs die and are replaced each second.

Each of the trillions of cells in the body can be likened to a walled city. Each "city" contains an administrative headquarters in the nucleus, with DNA serving as the city manager to guide and direct all activities. It contains active communication (RNA) and transport (endoplasmic reticulum) systems, power plants (mitochondria), factories (ribosomes), and an active waste disposal system (lysosomes). Oxygen and nutrients come in through the walls (cell membrane), and carbon dioxide and waste products are passed out through the walls.

The smallest functional units in the body are enzymes, the protein molecules which serve as workmen in the cell factories. Each enzyme performs only one function, but since a single cell may have more than one function, it may house hundreds or thousands of different enzymes. The RBC, compared to most cells, is very simple in that it has one principal product: hemoglobin.

The hemoglobin factory is schematically illustrated in Figure 4. The assembly line begins by (1) succinate and glycine joining to form porphobilinogen. This first step requires the use of three different enzymes plus vitamins and minerals. (2) Next, four of these molecules join to form protoporphyrin III with the help of six different enzymes and three vitamins. (3) Iron is added to protoporphyrin III to make heme by the action of one enzyme, one vitamin, and one mineral. (4) Finally, four molecules of heme attach to a molecule of globin, which has been produced separately, and hemoglobin rolls off the assembly line ready to serve its respiratory function.[7]

The complexity of enzyme activity is put in perspective when we realize that the comparatively simple hemoglobin assembly line uses 10 different enzymes, six vitamins, and four minerals to produce each molecule of hemoglobin. When it is further recognized that the body must produce three million new RBCs each second to replace those that die, and that each RBC contains almost 300 million molecules of hemoglobin, each made up of 10,000 atoms and 570 different amino acids, we begin to feel mind-boggled.[8] And remember, this is one of the simplest cells in the body. If we attempted to illustrate with liver or kidney cells, the complexity would be much greater.

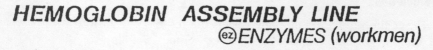

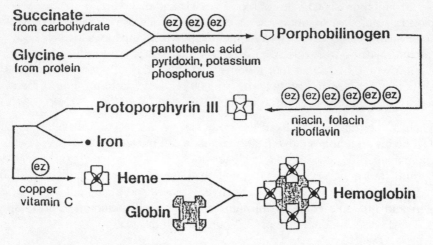

Figure 4. *Succinate and glycine combine (with the aid of three enzymes, two vitamins, and two minerals) to form porphobilinogen. Then four molecules of porphobilinogen are arranged (with the help of six enzymes and three vitamins) into a molecule of protoporphyrin III. An atom of iron is added (with the help of an enzyme, plus copper and vitamin C) to form heme. A molecule of globin arrives from another assembly line, and four molecules of heme attach themselves to it, forming a molecule of hemoglobin.*

These glimpses of God's design inspire awe and respect (reverent fear) for our Creator. The God who created us also created within us the laws of health. We show our love of God by our attitude toward His laws, both physical and spiritual. In reverent fear of our Creator, we eagerly desire to keep all His laws. The first angel seeks to arouse this attitude in humans as he urges preparation for the Second Coming.

---

[1] Revelation 14:7.

[2] Psalm 111:10.

[3] Exodus 34:6.

[4] Colin Mitchell, *The Case for Creationism* (Autumn House Limited, 1994) 138-140.

[5] Richard M. Ritland, *A Search for Meaning in Nature* (Pacific Press, 1970) 283-285.

[6] J. D. Ratcliff, "Bloodstream," *I Am Joe's Body* (A Berkley/ Reader's Digest Book, 1975) 89.

[7] Mervyn G. Hardinge, "Health and Salvation," *Journal of the Adventist Theological Society* 2 Mar. 1992: 94-110.

[8] *The Incredible Machine* (National Geographic Society, 1986) 100.

CHAPTER THREE

Give Glory and Worship

AND GIVE GLORY TO HIM . . . AND WORSHIP HIM WHO MADE HEAVEN AND EARTH, THE SEA AND SPRINGS OF WATER. REVELATION 14:7.

After admonishing us to "Fear God," the first angel instructs us to "give glory to Him."[1] How do we give glory to God? Paul answers this specifically in his letter to the Corinthians:

Do you not know that your body is the temple of the Holy Spirit, who is in you, whom you have from God, and you are not your own? For you were bought at a price; therefore glorify God *in your body* and in your spirit, which are God's.[2]

Paul had spoken before of the importance of our body temples: "Do you not know that you are the temple of God and that the Spirit of God dwells in you? If anyone defiles the temple of God, God will destroy him. For the temple of God is holy, which temple you are."[3] Paul further elaborates, "Therefore, whether you eat or drink, or whatever you do, do all to the glory of God."[4]

Scripture makes it clear that God intends for us to glorify Him with godly lifestyles, especially as we prepare for His second coming. Paul wrote to Titus that

the grace of God that brings salvation has appeared to all men, teaching us that, denying ungodliness and worldly lusts, we should *live soberly, right- eously, and godly* in this present age, looking for the blessed hope and glorious appearing of our great God and Savior Jesus Christ, who gave Himself for us, that He might redeem us from every lawless deed and purify for Himself His own special people, zealous for good works.[5]

We who are looking for the "blessed hope" of Christ's soon coming should be a special people in the pure lives we live. To the Thessalonians Paul gives this chal- lenge:

Now may the God of peace Himself sanctify you completely; and may your whole spirit, soul, *and body* be preserved blameless at the coming of our Lord Jesus Christ.[6]

Complete sanctification of body, soul, and spirit, by His grace, is needed for those who await Christ's coming. This type of living gives "glory to God."

To glorify God in our bodies means to take the best possible care of the bodies He gave us. They are His both by fact of (1) His creation of us and (2) His redemption of us. We can confidently look to Him—Designer, Creator, Lover, Redeemer—for instruction on how best to maintain life and health.

A parable illustrates this point.

Parable of the Automobile

An auto manufacturer decided to promote his products by loaning them to a few individuals who would demonstrate their beauty and value to other people. Two men gladly accepted this offer, and each was given a shiny new vehicle, along with an instruction manual on how to care for the car. The only requirement was that they take every opportunity to demonstrate to others the benefits of the vehicle, giving credit to the manufacturer.

The first man happily drove his new car home, but from the beginning was negligent in its care. He took no interest in keeping it clean, so soon it became dirty. There was no maintenance schedule for oil change and lubrication. Regular leaded gasoline was used despite the clear instructions to use only unleaded fuel. This first car quickly began to look and drive like a wreck.

By contrast, the second man took great pride in his new car. He cleaned and shined it daily. He faithfully followed directions for preventive maintenance, recognizing that the manufacturer knew best how to take care of the car. Only the highest quality fuel went into the gas tank. As well as possible, this man avoided accidents. Friends came to admire the vehicle's great performance, and many sought to obtain such a car for themselves.

When the loan period ended, the manufacturer visited each man to whom he had loaned a vehicle. He took the vehicle away from the first man and expressed deep disappointment in the way it had been cared for and in the lack of interest neighbors showed in the manufacturer. As he visited with the second man, the manufacturer became very pleased. The second man had shown respect for the manufacturer by caring for the vehicle well. Gladly the manufacturer renewed the contract with the second man and continued to provide him with a "demonstrator" vehicle.

The man who did not take good care of his borrowed car lost what he had. The one who had been conscientious was counted as a good steward and blessed with continued use of the vehicle. The second man had glorified the manufacturer.

Health and Ecology

Many people today worry about the steadily increasing cost of health care. Preventive medicine is gaining popularity because of its potential to reduce costs. In the ordinary practice of medicine, there is little incentive to bring costs down.

In many situations medical care has become very sophisticated and depersonalized. It has become big business, and health-care providers are no longer respected as the compassionate caregivers they once were. While the engineering approach in medicine has been useful, it is increasingly clear that simply removing or replacing defective body parts or attempting to destroy all germs is not sufficient or ecologically sound. A better approach is one which aims to build up a person's own immune system with an improved lifestyle.

Ecology is a philosophy of medical practice, not just an environmental issue. Historian Alan Gregg has divided medical history into three major eras:

1. The era of **authority**—from antiquity to the beginning of modern medical science in the 1800s.

2. The era of **research, experimentation, and treatment of specific diseases**—from the nineteenth century to now.

3. The era of **ecology**, just now beginning, in which the focus of medical attention becomes the whole patient and his environment rather than just disease.

Gregg points out that "many of the current problems in public health and medical care spring from the difficulties of this period of transition."[7]

The ecologic view suggests that humans and their interactions with the environment must be changed. Stanley Cobb states,

The behavior of the living organism, as a whole or in its parts, has now become the focus of interest of biologists and, somewhat more tardily, of physicians. They are beginning to conceive of both health and disease as reactions of the human organism to a complex internal and external environment. . . . At long last, the ecological point of view is pervading modern medicine.[8]

Throughout history humans have vacillated between blaming sickness and disease on outside forces and blaming themselves. Just over a hundred years ago when Pasteur demonstrated the germ theory, the question seemed to have been decisively settled in favor of disease being the result of hostile outside forces. Modern medicine has been built largely on the belief that attacking outside forces is more important than trying to change people.

With this philosophy we invest in the development of new antibiotics to fight increasingly resistant organisms; meanwhile, in the psychological realm, we try to alter the moral code of society to alleviate guilt and stress. A common attitude is that human health habits need not, or cannot, change. The emphasis in medical treatment is mostly on what health professionals do *to people*. What people do *for themselves* to prevent or treat sickness is considered less important.

Rene Dubos reminds us that we are actually creating new diseases for ourselves as rapidly as we subdue old ones.[9] Physicians could help alleviate this problem by influencing people to change instead of by compounding the problem by fighting diseases which are quickly supplanted by other diseases.

Health Reform

Another serious problem exists in the United States and has received great publicity in the media. The annual costs of health care now exceed $3,000 for each man, woman, and child in the nation. Health care accounts for about 13 percent of the gross national product, far more than in any other country. Several countries, however, have better statistics in longevity or infant mortality than does the U.S. This suggests there may be ways to more efficiently provide health care. It also indicates a lack of direct relationship between the cost and effectiveness of health care. Less costly approaches can be effective.

In many industries, employee health care is the single greatest expense. In the automobile industry, the cost of employee health care per vehicle manufactured is now more than the value of the steel used in the vehicle! These high costs fuel the demand for reform. *Health reform*, in this context, refers to the effort to reduce or prevent the continued rise of health costs in the United States.

In the early 1970s Canada recognized its own problem and instituted a monumental study to get at the roots of the issue. By identifying the principal causes of sickness and death, the Canadian government developed what it called the **Health Field Concept.** This framework for looking at health consists of four elements:

Human biology. This embraces all aspects of health which develop within the body as a result of basic human biology and genetic inheritance.

Environment. This includes all conditions outside the body that affect health and over which humans usually have little control. These include unsafe or contaminated food, drugs, and cosmetics; air, noise, and water pollution; and other health hazards.

Lifestyle. This consists of the choices made by individuals in areas over which they have some degree of control. These include decisions about how, when, and what an individual eats or drinks; his exercise and rest habits; and a myriad of other choices that affects one's risk of disease or health. Self-assumed risks lead, for example, to "diseases of choice" such as emphysema, lung cancer, or heart disease for those who choose to smoke; or cirrhosis of the liver or auto accidents for those who choose to drink alcohol.

Health-care organization. This refers to the workers, facilities, and equipment known as the "health-care system." Traditionally, 95 cents of every health dollar spent—virtually all the resources and attention—go to this one element. Although consuming the majority of resources, the health-care system, with all its doctors and hospitals, is relatively helpless to prevent disease or promote health.

In taking this approach to the elements affecting health, the Canadian study makes clear that

improvements in health now depend far more on how we behave as individuals, on our life-style, than on improvements in the quality or quantity of health care. The individual's health is now largely in his own hands. If fortunate to be born free of congenital disease, an individual by controlling his behavior, can do more to preserve his health and to extend his life than can be achieved by specific preventive or therapeutic medicine.[10]

This concept has been confirmed in many other countries. Risk assessment and lifestyle education are potent new tools which originated with this concept. People must learn that the lifestyle they choose to follow largely determines their level of health and their quality of life.

Also, it needs to be understood that much health education is wasted by assuming all people have the same felt needs. **Risk assessment** attempts to categorize people according to their individual risks of specific disease. For instance, individuals with elevated blood cholesterol who live sedentary lives, smoke cigarettes, and have a family history of heart disease have a very high risk of heart attack. When this risk is understood, people feel the need to decrease their risk and will listen much more seriously to health education than those who do not know their risk. A **felt need** comes either from desire to alleviate existing pain or illness or from recognition of individual risk factors that seriously predispose to disease.

Choose Life

Inherent in the concept of lifestyle and risk avoidance is the idea that human beings have choice. God gave humans this wonderful gift in the beginning. He never uses force, but He does urge us to make good choices. As Moses gave his last message on behalf of God to the Israelites, he pled, "*choose life*, that both you and your descendants may live."[11]

Notice the last words of Moses before he climbed Mount Nebo to die:

Set your hearts on all the words which I testify among you today, which you shall command your children to be careful to observe—all the words of this law. For it is not a futile (vain) thing for you, because it is your life, and by this word you shall *prolong your days* in the land which you cross over the Jordan to possess.[12]

God emphasizes the relationship of cause and effect. If we live according to His commands, then the natural result is life and health. Disobedience brings a natural result of disease and death.

Several years later Joshua gave this last testament to the children of Israel:

If it seems evil to you to serve the Lord, choose for yourselves this day whom you will serve . . . but as for me and my house, we will serve the Lord.[13]

Giving glory to God in our bodies includes making good choices. "Choose life!" was the plea of Moses. It remains God's call to us by the first angel.

---

[1] Revelation 14:7.

[2] 1 Corinthians 6:19, 20.

[3] 1 Corinthians 3:16, 17.

[4] 1 Corinthians 10:31.

[5] Titus 2:11-14.

[6] 1 Thessalonians 5:23, 24.

[7] Edward A. Suchman, ed., *Sociology and the Field of Public Health* (Russell Sage Foundation, New York) 18.

[8] Harold I. Lief, F. Victor, and R. Nino, eds., *The Psychological Basis of Medical Practice* (Harper and Row) 37.

[9] Rene J. Dubos, *Mirage of Health* (New York: Harper).

[10] From an address by the Honorable Marc LaLonde, Minister of National Health and Welfare of Canada, to the First Pan American Conference on Health Manpower Planning, Ottawa, Canada, 10-14 September 1973.

[11] Deuteronomy 30:19.

[12] Deuteronomy 32:46, 47.

[13] Joshua 24:15.

CHAPTER FOUR

Eat to the Glory of God

EAT . . . TO THE GLORY OF GOD. 1 CORINTHIANS 10:31.

The first angel of Revelation 14 says, "Fear God and give glory to Him. . . ."[1] Paul makes it clear that we should eat "to the glory of God."[2] What we eat is vital to the development and maintenance of our body temples. Our strength, our level of immunity, and our very existence and ability to contribute to society depend on an adequate diet. We glorify God in the way we provide nourishment to our bodies, His temples. What is God's plan for an optimum diet?

Nutrition Science

Nutrition as a science is relatively new. It originated with the Frenchman Antoine Lavoisier, who earned his title as the father of modern nutrition when he recognized in the late eighteenth century that "life is a chemical function."[3] He particularly recognized the relation between oxygen and food metabolism.

But not until recently has information on specific nutrients been compiled. Vitamins, for instance, were first isolated by such pioneers as Casimir Funk in Poland, F. G. Hopkins in Great Britain, and Elmer V. McCollum, Joseph Goldberger, and Robert R. Williams in the U.S. during the early twentieth century.[4]

In 1753 Scottish naval surgeon James Lind published the results of the first scientifically controlled therapeutic study in humans. It showed that scurvy—a serious deficiency disease manifested by swollen gums, hemorrhage, and weakness—could be cured by citrus fruit. This was the first disease for which a specific cure was discovered. The subsequent requirement that all British sailors take a regular ration of citrus juice led to their nickname as "limeys." It took almost 200 years, however, for ascorbic acid (vitamin C) to be isolated and for this preventive measure to become generally accepted. We continue to learn more about this and other nutrients daily.[5]

Nutrition can only be understood as we begin to comprehend the function of body cells. Each of the trillions of cells in our bodies continues its work night and day. Each cell requires fuel (food), which is most efficiently obtained from starchy foods (hydrocarbons) that are metabolized (burned) in the presence of oxygen (from respiration). Fat can be a source of energy or stored calories, and it is also vital for the production of certain hormones and the maintenance of cell walls. Substances containing nitrogen (amino acids) are important in forming the structure of the cell and its enzymes. Vitamins are required in minute amounts by metabolic processes in the body, frequently in association with enzymes. Both vitamins and minerals are facilitators of enzyme chemical reactions.

Nutrition is the science of providing all the basic nutrients (vitamins, minerals, water, enzymes, hydrocarbons, amino acids, and fats) needed for each cell all the time. The body is remarkably able to recover and reuse almost all nutrients from the body's constantly dying cells. Because of this efficient recovery system, most nutrients, especially vitamins and minerals, are needed daily only in microscopic amounts.

Foods

The practical approach to nutrition is not the study of chemistry but a recognition of the proper intake of foods needed to preserve health. Whole foods, prepared as simply as possible, provide the most nutritious diet.

The original diet given in Eden is outlined in Genesis:

See, I have given you *every herb that yields seed* which is on the face of all the earth, *and every tree whose fruit yields seed*; to you it shall be for food.[6]

The curse after sin suggested an addition to the original diet. This was stated to Adam as follows:

Cursed is the ground for your sake; in toil you shall eat of it all the days of your life. Both thorns and thistles it shall bring forth for you, and you shall eat *the herb of the field*.[7]

To the original diet of grains, legumes, fruits, and nuts was added green leafy vegetables and roots such as potatoes and carrots (the herb of the field).

This diet sustained life remarkably well. Prior to the flood there was no evidence of decreasing longevity. Jared, Methuselah, and Noah (the sixth, eighth, and tenth generations from Adam) lived longer than Adam himself.[8]

After the flood destroyed the earth and its vegetation, God suggested an alternative diet:

Every moving thing that lives shall be food for you. I have given you all things, even as the green herbs. But you shall not eat flesh with its life, that is, its blood.[9]

The restriction against eating blood was further amplified to the Israelites as they prepared to enter the Promised Land: "This shall be a *perpetual* statute throughout your generations in all your dwellings: you shall *eat neither fat nor blood.*"[10] This suggests a permanent dietary restriction designed for humanity's continuing health. What a difference it would make today if people ate their meat without fat or blood.

Life Span of Man Before and After the Flood
Primarily from Genesis 5 and Genesis 11

10 Generations Before the Flood		10 Generations After the Flood	
Name	**Age at Death in Years**	**Name**	**Age at Death in Years**
1. Adam	930	1. Shem	600
2. Seth	912	2. Arphaxad	438
3. Enosh	905	3. Salah	433
4. Cainan	910	4. Eber	464
5. Mahalalel	895	5. Peleg	238
6. Jared	962	6. Reu	239
7. Enoch (translated)	365+	7. Serug	230
8. Methuselah	969	8. Nahor	148
9. Lamech	777	9. Terah	205
10. Noah	950	10. Abraham	175
Average life span (discounting Enoch)	912.2	Average life span	317

Figure 5. *The ages of the 10 generations who ate vegetarian diets before the flood compared with the 10 generations who began eating animals for food after the flood.*

That flesh food was intended to cut short sinful lives is not stated, but the results recorded in Genesis 11 and 12 are dramatic. Following the flood, life spans rapidly declined. Abraham, the tenth from Noah, lived 175 years. This contrasts with Noah, the tenth from Adam, who lived 950 years, 20 years longer than Adam himself.[11]

Scientists increasingly prove that the original diet is the best kind for preventing heart attacks and strokes and for controlling diabetes, many kinds of cancer, hypertension, arthritis, obesity, diverticulitis, and kidney stones—all of which are now common in Western populations. The animal fat and cholesterol in meat, eggs, and milk are major culprits. High fiber, phytochemicals, antioxidants, and readily available essential vitamins and minerals are just a few of the additional benefits of the original plant-based diet of Eden.

In 1983 The China Study began to do a cross-sectional survey of diet, lifestyle, and disease mortality characteristics of 6,500 adults in 130 villages of rural China. Dr. T. Colin Campbell, the principal investigator in the study, has come to a new hypothesis. Rather than assuming that dietary fat is the chief cause of degenerative disease, a better hypothesis says that an improper balance between animal and plant foods is the chief cause. He says there are "overwhelmingly compelling observations that suggest that the nutritional characteristics of foods of animal origin enhance degenerative diseases, whereas the nutritional characteristics of foods of plant origin inhibit the development of these diseases." Although increased consumption of fruits, vegetables, and grains is now widely recommended, he suggests there is not sufficient emphasis put on decreased consumption of foods of animal origin. Because of commercial pressure, attempts are made to "preserve the traditional intake of animal foods" by swapping, for example, chicken for beef or low-fat for whole-fat dairy products, giving a false sense of confidence in the value of low-fat animal foods.[12]

The China Study points out that the Chinese have much less heart disease, cancer, osteoporosis, and iron-deficiency anemia than the U.S. population. This is despite the fact that 96 percent of Chinese protein comes from plant foods. In the U.S., 71 percent of protein intake comes from animal sources.[13] Since all nutrients originate in plants, it is unfortunate that so many people choose to obtain their nutrients secondhand through animals.

Dr. Dean Ornish, the respected cardiologist who has demonstrated the reversibility of atherosclerotic coronary heart disease, has developed what he calls the *Life Choice* diet. Ornish emphasizes foods low in fat but high in complex carbohydrates (starches), fiber, and other nutrients found only in plant foods. He recommends avoiding meat of all kinds, including chicken and fish.[14]

Summarizing an immense amount of nutritional research, Dr. Mark Messina, a research scientist and nutritionist formerly with the National Cancer Institutes, says,

Eat lots of whole grains, vegetables, and fruits. Include some soy or other beans in your diet every day. Use only tiny amounts of nuts, seeds, fats, and animal foods, or skip them if you prefer. Believe it or not, this is all you really need to know.[15]

John A. McDougall has published the widely accepted McDougall Plan. In it he writes,

Rich foods are so common that people forget that not long ago they were served as delicacies, and then only to the wealthy classes. . . . 'Rich' foods include red meat, poultry, eggs, fish, shellfish, cheeses, milk, oils, nuts, seeds, white rice, refined flour, processed foods, salt, and sugar. . . . From a nutritional viewpoint, rich foods are those that provide poorly for our bodily needs because of either deficiencies or harmful excesses.

McDougall summarizes by saying,

> The diet that best supports health and healing for humans is a pure vegetable diet centered around starch foods with the addition of fresh fruits and vegetables.[16]

Scientific evidence supporting a plant diet is overwhelming. The myths associated with concern for adequate protein and the need for meat and dairy foods are increasingly recognized as propaganda from the influential meat and dairy industries. These industries invested heavily in new university departments of nutrition in the early twentieth century. Due to their influence, nutrition education from its beginning was biased. This bias toward meat and dairy is still voiced by some out-of-date nutrition counselors.

The relationship of poor diet to an increase in Western degenerative diseases is now being felt in the developing countries of Africa, Asia, and Latin America. As they follow the Western example of a diet high in animal products, heart and other degenerative diseases increase. Burkitt points out that

> the best example of significantly lower rates in the case of many, if not most, Western diseases are the *Seventh-Day Adventists* [sic], who, besides being largely vegetarian, are also nonsmokers with a low consumption of alcohol. They have been shown to have much lower rates of coronary heart disease, diabetes, cerebrovascular disease (strokes), and renal stones. Moreover, they suffer less from several cancers common in Western countries (lung and colon in men; lung, breast, and colon in women).[17]

To the extent that Adventists have followed the original diet of Eden, they have been blessed.

Food Ecology

Peter Burwash characterizes eating meat as an "ecological crime." An old Buddhist proverb says, "The frog does not drink up the pond in which he lives."[18] Unfortunately, food supplies are running out.

World Watch calculated in September, 1995, that "measured in days of global consumption, the world's estimated carryover stocks of grain for 1996 had fallen to 49 days—the lowest level ever recorded." Today only a handful of countries are able to consistently export grain: Argentina, Australia, Canada, France, and the United States. In 1995 U.S. grain made up nearly one-half of all international grain exports. *World Watch* reports, "Already, the 94 million [persons] being added to the global population each year are being fed only by reducing the consumption of those already here."[19] This means that many of the world's poorest, who are now spending most of their meager incomes on just enough food to survive, may not make it to the next harvest.

It has been assumed during food shortages that farmers could always bring more land into cultivation. This is no longer true. Available land which is not too cold, dry, steep, or barren is nearly all in cultivation. Much of it is degraded by topsoil depletion and erosion and must be taken out of cultivation at some point. The annual rate of soil erosion in the U.S. is an estimated 27 tons per hectare (one hectare equals 2.47 acres). In developing countries, erosion rates are probably twice that much. Because so much unproductive land has been taken out of cultivation, the grain harvest area in the former Soviet Union shrank from 123 million to 94 million hectares between 1977 and 1994.[20] Other land around the world is lost to urbanization, industrialization, and highways.

In addition, water tables are falling in many farming regions. In the Great Plains of the U.S., farmers have been forced since 1982 to decrease irrigation. Water tables in India are falling in several states, including the country's breadbasket, the Punjab. In China, much of the northern region suffers from water deficits. Around Beijing, the water table has dropped from 15 feet below ground in 1950 to more than 150 feet below ground in 1995.

Many rivers have been tapped, diverted, and dammed until little water is left to run into the sea. In 1995, China's Yellow River completely disappeared some 620 kilometers from its mouth on the Yellow Sea. The Colorado River in the U.S. has disappeared in the Arizona desert since 1993, rarely ever reaching the Gulf of California. In Central Asia, the Amu Darya is drained by cotton farmers before it reaches the Aral Sea, resulting in the loss of a large fishery business.[21] How true it is of our world today that "the whole land is made desolate, because no one takes it to heart [cares]."[22]

Until the 1980s agricultural production could always be expanded by increased use of fertilizers. In 1990 the world passed a little-noticed but fateful turning point in human history. Though it worked superbly for half a century, farmers have found that increasing crop yields by adding more and more fertilizer is like a baker adding more and more yeast to the dough. After tripling from 1950 to 1990, world grain production has not gained at all since 1990, largely because crops cannot effectively use more fertilizer. It is questionable whether plant breeders can solve the food crisis by developing new varieties that can increase production through use of more fertilizers.[23] The stage seems set for the "famines and pestilences" prophesied in Matthew.[24]

Jules Verne long ago suggested that when we reach the limits of food production on land, we can turn to the oceans. Many countries have already done this. Between 1950 and 1989, the world fish catch expanded more than fourfold to 100 million tons annually. The United Nations calculates that the world, because of overfishing, reached its limits in 1989. The fish catch has declined about 8 percent since that year, and the world now faces declining seafood per person and rising seafood prices.[25]

How does meat eating relate to the ecological crisis? Very simply. Forty percent of the world's grain goes to feed animals for meat production. (In the U.S., 70 percent of grain and millions of tons of soybeans go to feed animals.) If these products were consumed directly by humans, five times more people could be nourished.[26] Vegetarian food requires less than one-third the energy to produce as does a similar quantity of meat. Nearly seven pounds of corn and soy are needed to put one pound of boneless, trimmed pork on the table in the United States.[27]

In 1977 the energy input of U.S. food production was calculated. Producing, processing, distributing, and preparing a one-pound can of sweet corn providing 375 kilocalories (kcal) of food energy required 4,100 kcal of production energy. To produce 375 kcal of food energy from beef required 19,990 kcal—nearly five times more.

Simpler agricultural techniques also have their costs. In Mexico, where the "cut-and-burn" maize culture was investigated, a total of 1,144 hours of labor was required to grow a hectare of maize (corn). This provided an annual food supply for seven people eating primarily grains and vegetables—2,700 kcal per person daily. If, instead of this vegetarian diet, the family of seven consumed the animal-based diet preferred in the U.S., about 5,000 hours of labor would be required to feed them for a year.[28]

Just the water needed to supply Americans with meat comes to about 190 gallons per person per day, or twice what typical Americans use at home for all purposes each day.[29] Livestock production is the most ecologically damaging part of American agriculture. Unfortunately, every nation in the world that is wealthy enough seems to be taking notes from the United States and is starting to shower resources on the meat industry. American-style animal farms seem to be the wave of the future.[30] The prospect of 6 billion people eating the way Americans do is an ecological impossibility. Eating like Americans would require 2.5 times more grain than the world can grow.[31] The only practical solution is for all people to shift their consumption to more healthy and less costly plant foods.

The widespread ecological consequences of animal production are just beginning to appear. Although the United States produces most of its own food, its meat appetite is so great that it also imports beef from Latin America. Cost Rica, for example, was once nearly covered by tropical forest. By 1983, after two decades of explosive growth in the cattle industry, only 17 percent of the original forest remained; the rest had been cut for cattle grazing. It is calculated that a single hamburger from Costa Rica involves the destruction of 55 square feet of rain forest. Clearing this much land releases up to 165 pounds of carbon dioxide, the "greenhouse" gas that is changing the global environment.[32]

Rain forests are the lungs of our planet, producing oxygen and using up carbon dioxide. Cattle ranchers are burning more than 27 million acres of rain forest in the Amazon basin annually. The destruction of rain forests in South America helps cause the climatic changes which increase the growth of deserts in Africa. These rain forests also provide winter homes to thousands of migratory birds from North America. Many birds die due to lost homes, meaning that fewer birds return northward to control insects. The increase of insects requires more insecticides, which pollute land and water and ultimately get into the sea. Fish contaminated by insecticides have been found in all oceans, including both the Arctic and Antarctic oceans.[33]

These numerous problems help show why concern for the environment is one of the most common reasons for being a vegetarian today. The moral/ethical issues related to the unnecessary taking of life and the economic and environmental issues related to animal foods are sufficient to justify vegetarianism. Looming ever larger, however, is the serious ethical question of whether it is right for people to eat flesh food if, by eating it, they are depriving others of having any food at all. If the world can provide five times as much food through plant sources as through animal sources, can we condone the habits of a few wealthy people who desire meat? Meat eating uses up resources that might enable starving people to survive.

All of this ignores the basic health problems associated with eating meat—high saturated fat, high cholesterol, low fiber, naturally occurring urea and other wastes, and often antibiotics, hormones, bacterial and viral infections, or parasites. All of these health hazards should give a meat eater reason to pause. The benefits of God's original plant-based diet are overwhelming when compared to animal-based food.

Antioxidants

One of the most important elements for life is oxygen. Every cell of the body requires it for energy metabolism. Deprived of oxygen, a cell will die in seconds. Oxygen helps provide energy in the body by burning fuel (food) to power the activity of every cell and, therefore, all functions of the body.

For some years we have recognized that in addition to regular oxygen, we also find in the body unstable oxygen, commonly known as "free radicals." Chemical stability occurs in a molecule when all atomic electrons are matched. Free radicals have an unbalanced number of electrons and aggressively seek to join with or "oxidize" other molecules, acting in many ways like a magnet toward other molecules. Free radicals have been referred to as "cellular wrecking crews."[34]

In small amounts free radicals are good to kill bacteria, fight inflammation, and control the tone of the smooth muscles in blood vessels. In larger numbers, however, free radicals directly damage DNA and thereby promote cancer, especially in sites such as the lungs, cervix, skin, stomach, prostate, colon, and esophagus. They are strongly implicated in the blood vessel damage that leads to plaque formation and atherosclerosis (the deposit of cholesterol in blood vessel walls).

Free radicals also severely damage the immune system by their effect on white blood cells. The ill effects of free radicals are evident in the aging process, including the breakdown and sagging of skin tissues. In fact, free radicals have been implicated in more than fifty diseases, including such diverse problems as cataracts, Parkinson's disease, and brain hemorrhage in premature infants.[35]

Fortunately the body is designed to take care of a few free radicals by its normally produced endogenous (internally produced) antioxidants, which quickly subdue small numbers of free radicals. The best-known natural antioxidant enzymes include superoxide dismutase (SOD), catalase, and glutathione peroxidase (GSH). These are constantly working to protect us.

Factors that lead to excess free radicals include these:

- intake of too many oxidants, such as fat and iron (as in meat)
- breathing polluted air, especially cigarette smoke
- overexposure to ultraviolet light (from the sun)
- some pesticides, certain drugs, and chemical contaminants of foods and drinks
- excessive amounts of exercise—excessive in time and/or effort
- uncontrolled diabetes and its high levels of blood sugar
- emotional stress
- radiation (x-rays or cosmic rays from space)
- reperfusion—the return of blood to an organ temporarily deprived (similar to reperfusion is the shunting of blood from the muscles and other organs to the stomach after eating a heavy meal)
- asbestos and other irritating fibers or particles that enter the lungs [36]

Dr. Kenneth Cooper, founder of the aerobics movement, is now promoting what he calls the "antioxidant revolution." It includes these practices:

1. low-intensity exercise, such as walking (in contrast to running), to minimize your output of injurious free radicals and stimulate production of natural antioxidants
2. intake of fruits and vegetables prepared in ways that maximize their antioxidant effects
3. avoidance of environmental factors known to stimulate excess free radical formation
4. daily intake of the major antioxidants nutrients: vitamin E, beta-carotene, vitamin C
   - Vitamin E occurs naturally in almonds, sunflower seeds, sweet potatoes, whole wheat, wheat germ, and most vegetable oils. (Natural vitamin E extracted from vegetable oils is *d-alpha tocopherol*. Less helpful is the synthetic vitamin E, *dl-alpha tocopherol*.)
   - Beta carotene occurs in the yellow-orange and dark green vegeta-

bles and fruits: kale, chard, spinach, carrots, pumpkins, sweet potatoes, tomatoes, squash, broccoli, cantaloupe, apricots, mangos, and
papayas. (Please note that the fully formed vitamin A, found in liver,
butter, and eggs, does not have an antioxidant effect and is toxic in
large doses.)
- Vitamin C is abundant in all fruits, berries, and melons. Especially
  good sources are citrus fruits and cruciferous and dark green leafy
  vegetables.[37]

Other antioxidants include selenium and Probucol, which are not recommended as routine supplements. Except for vitamin E, recommended amounts of
the antioxidants listed above can be found easily in foods. Sufficient vitamin E from
food may require a higher fat intake than is usually recommended. As a strong
believer in obtaining nutrients from food, I do not endorse daily supplements.[38]
Let's avoid the temptation to obtain nutrients artificially.

Another reason to act cautiously in taking routine food supplements is the fact
that the body has a tendency to adapt to its usual intake of nutrients. Take calcium,
for example. People who become used to a high calcium intake, as do most
Westerners, adapt so that they require high intake of calcium to prevent calcium
deficiency. People in most of the developing world live with a low calcium intake
and have no problem maintaining their blood calcium levels; in fact, they have
much less osteoporosis than do Americans. Once a person has adapted to high
intakes, it can be difficult to readapt to lower intakes. Why force our bodies to
adapt to high levels of any nutrient and thereby make ourselves more dependent
on that nutrient?

Phytochemicals

Phytochemicals (plant chemicals), components of foods that are not nutrients
but do affect health, are causing lots of excitement in the scientific world. Some
suggest that recognition of vitamins in the early twentieth century caused the first
dietary revolution; the recognition of the anticancer phytochemicals is now
ushering in the second golden age of nutrition. Beginning in the 1980s, it was
increasingly recognized in many studies that people who eat lots of fruits and
vegetables have a lower cancer risk. The National Cancer Institute and the National
Academy of Sciences began at that time to recommend increased consumption of
fruits and vegetables, especially cruciferous vegetables—cabbage, broccoli, brussel
sprouts, cauliflower, kale, collards, mustard greens, rutabagas, radishes, and
turnips. (These cancer-fighting vegetables take their name from the Latin word for
cross because they bear cross-shaped flowers.)

Multiple studies show how potent phytochemicals are in the fight against
cancer and other diseases. Early attention focused on the pigments that give plants
their color. The best-known plant pigment is beta-carotene, one of more than five

hundred different carotenoids, many of which have been shown to be powerful fighters against disease. Quite a fad developed in recent years of providing beta-carotene supplements, but studies now seem to confirm that the benefits of the foods are not available from beta-carotene in tablet form.[39]

Other phytochemical classes and their food sources include these:

- Coumarins—vegetables and citrus fruits
- Allium compounds—onions, garlic, and chives
- Dithiolthiones—cruciferous vegetables
- Flavonoids—most fruits and vegetables
- Glucosinolates—cruciferous vegetables
- Glyceritinic acid—licorice
- Inositol hexaphosphate—particularly in soybeans and cereals
- Isoflavones—soybeans
- Isothiocyanates, thiocyanates—cruciferous vegetables
- Lignans—flax seeds
- Limonene—citrus fruits
- Phenols—most fruits and vegetables
- Plant sterols—vegetables, including soybeans
- Protease inhibitors—most plants, particularly seeds and legumes such as soybeans
- Saponins—plants, particularly soybeans[40]

Each of these phytochemical classes contains many compounds. For instance, isoflavones, perhaps the best of the anticarcinogens, contain both equol, an antiestrogenic substance, and genistein. These together protect against a number of cancers, including breast, colon, lung, prostate, skin, and leukemia. Soybeans are the only commonly consumed food containing significant amounts of isoflavones.[41]

Speaking of soybeans, few foods have so much going for them. Soybeans are high in fiber and rich in high-quality protein, calcium, iron, zinc, and many of the B vitamins. They are relatively high in fat when compared to other plants, but it is unsaturated fat, and the level is lower than in most animal products. About 50 percent of the fat in soy oil is linoleic acid, a polyunsaturated fat. As with all plants, soybeans contain no cholesterol. New information indicates they are rich in phytochemicals (which fight cancer) and are more effective in lowering blood cholesterol than oat bran.

Studies show that all dietary fiber slows the release of glucose into the bloodstream and makes cells more sensitive to insulin, thus helping to control diabetes. Soy fiber works effectively in this. A University of Texas study showed that humans who had protein from meat and dairy foods lost 50 percent more calcium from their bodies that did those who had only soy protein. This suggests that soy also protects against osteoporosis. High protein intake harms the kidneys, but a British study found the filtration rate (a measure of how hard the kidneys have to work to get rid of waste products such as ammonia) was 16 percent higher after a meal of animal protein than it was after a meal of soy protein. Other studies show that both kidney stones and gallstones occur twice as often in meat eaters as in vegetarians. The health benefits of plant foods, soybeans in particular, go on and on.[42]

About half the world's soybeans are grown the U.S. But instead of eating soybeans, Americans either feed them to animals or export them. About one-third of American soybeans are exported to countries such as Japan, where they are a dietary staple—and where heart attacks, cancer, osteoporosis, and iron-deficiency anemia are lower than in the U.S. About 90 to 95 percent of the soybeans that stay in the country are fed to animals.[43] By not eating the soybeans directly, we are denying ourselves health advantages that can help fight cancer and heart disease. Meanwhile, eating meat from animals raised on those same soybeans increases our risk for disease.

One last note about beans. For some, beans are synonymous with gas. This is caused by complex sugars—stachyose, verbascose, and raffinose—which human enzymes cannot digest. However, hundreds of bacteria live in our colon, most of them beneficial to health. They help digest the complex sugars that our digestive enzymes cannot, but in the process produce gas: carbon dioxide, hydrogen, and sometimes methane.

One of these bacteria, bifidobacteria, appears to be especially helpful in the health of the colon and seems to prevent infections by harmful bacteria. In Japan, where it has been much studied, bifidobacteria has been shown to be related to longevity. People with a good number of bifidobacteria in their colon live considerably longer than those who have few or none. Whole soy beans, soy flour, and textured soy protein encourage the growth of bifidobacteria; tofu and the fermented soy products do not cause the growth of these helpful bacteria.[44]

For those troubled by bean gas, here are a few suggestions. First, eat beans in small quantities, preferably in combination with low-fat foods. Eat slowly, chewing food well. Avoid water and liquids with meals. Avoid eating beans with other gas-producing foods such as cabbage. Don't eat beans late at night. In preparing dry beans, soak them at least three hours, preferably changing the soaking water more than once. Discarding the soaking water before cooking helps remove some of the complex sugars. Be sure beans are thoroughly cooked before eating them. A new enzyme product called BEANO claims to prevent gas problems by making the indigestible sugars more digestible. Fortunately, for most people, flatulence is not a big problem and can be overcome with the suggestions above. The potential phytochemical benefits make it worth trying.

Empty Calories

Through Isaiah, God asks,

> Why do you spend money for what is not bread, and your wages for what does not satisfy? Listen carefully to Me, and eat what is good.[45]

Refined foods are excellent examples of wasting money for what is not real food but empty calories. Common sugar is a pure product made up of just the simple carbohydrate, sucrose. It contains not a single vitamin or mineral. Although easily digested and metabolized, it requires vitamins and minerals for metabolism and can, therefore, cause nutritional deficiencies by utilizing nutrients it doesn't contain (which have to be robbed from other foods or body stores).

Refined white bread is not much better. The milling and refining process removes 50 to 90 percent of nutrients from the wheat, including many amino acids (protein particles) and most of the vitamins and minerals, plus 75 percent of the fiber. In the U.S. white flour is required to be "enriched." The "enrichment" consists of returning portions of four of the more than 20 nutrients removed—iron and three of the B vitamins. How would you feel if someone took $20 from you and told you they were "enriching" you by giving you $4 back? "Enriched flour" is really impoverished flour.

Visible fats—oil, salad dressing, hydrogenated fats such as margarine and mayonnaise, and butter—are even worse examples of empty calories. They provide nine calories per gram (compared to four in sugar and other refined food) and have few, if any, nutrients. Excess calories lead to obesity and other health problems, in addition to potential metabolic deficiencies caused by the lack of nutrients in refined foods. In times past, much emphasis was put on the advantages of polyunsaturated fats (oils from plants) over saturated fats, which come almost entirely from animals. Today we simply recommend reducing all fat intake. Most people eat far too much fat.

Fast foods are a classic example of empty calories. Unfortunately, most people are either born with or cultivate appetites for refined foods, sweets, and fats. We demand butter or margarine on our bread (doubling the calories) or high-fat dressings or mayonnaise on our salads (frequently tripling or quadrupling the calories).

In contrast, high-density foods are those which contain the most essential nutrients per calorie or per serving. Most high-density foods are plant foods simply prepared and eaten whole. Cooked dark green leafy vegetables are perhaps the best recommended example. One good serving of dark green leafy vegetables to everyone each day could do more to improve the health of the world than almost anything. They are rich in iron and calcium and the antioxidant vitamins C, beta-carotene, and E. They also contain fiber and a small amount of high-quality protein, along with no cholesterol and essentially no fat. Eating such foods gives "glory to

God" and enables Him to more easily give us abundant health.

Nutritional Precautions and Suggestions

It is impossible, in one chapter, to cover the whole science of nutrition. In fact, there is the very real danger of an imbalanced presentation which overemphasizes certain points. In this section I hope to bring the nutrition presentation into a balanced perspective. A beautiful thing about nutrition is that it should be an applied science, in which results can be observed relatively soon. If dietary changes do not promote better health, then they are not good nutrition.

Daniel and his three friends are good examples of nutrition research scientists. They asked the steward who had been set over them to give them just a 10-day therapeutic trial of a simple plant-based diet. The results were positive: after 10 days they "appeared better and fatter in flesh than all the young men who ate the portion of the king's delicacies."[46] Experience has subsequently shown that 10 days to two weeks is minimally sufficient to allow for many dietary adjustments.

There are situations in which gradual changes are better; however, in many ways, a comprehensive change in diet and lifestyle is easier to bring about than many small or moderate changes. Small changes can make one feel deprived (and hungry) but are not enough to make one feel better. Comprehensive changes often result in one feeling better so quickly that the benefits become much more obvious. Most people are positive about changes if they can understand and feel the advantages.

The taste for fat and spices is acquired. People who have become used to rich, spicy foods often forget the delicate flavors of simple, uncontaminated food. If, for example, you change from a high-salt to a low-salt diet, the food seems tasteless at first, but in ten days to two weeks the adjustment occurs. Now normally salted food tastes too salty! If, however, you regularly or occasionally eat salty foods, then you never adjust to the good taste of food with less salt. This principle holds for all dietary changes.[47]

Nutrition is concerned not only with what one eats, but also how and when it is eaten. For many semi-sedentary people, the author included, two meals a day are preferable to three or more. It is important, as much as possible, to eat at regular times with at least five hours between meals and no snacks between meals. An exercise break is much more beneficial than a coffee/snack break in mid-morning or mid-afternoon. Breakfast, which prepares one for the day's activities, is the most important meal of the day. It is best to drink water at least one-half hour before meals or a couple hours after. Water with meals dilutes digestive juices and interferes with metabolism. Food should be eaten slowly enough to relish its taste, chewed well, and eaten in a comfortable, pleasant environment. Light exercise after eating aids digestion; heavy exercise stops digestion. The last meal of the day should be taken several hours before retiring. Such practices are easy to try; your body will confirm whether they are good for you or not.

Simplify your food selection by learning to build each meal around a complex carbohydrate, the body's preferred energy source. This is frequently a local staple starchy food. While it is good to eat a variety of foods, it is best not to have too many varieties at one meal. Sometimes the staple may be potato; at other times, rice, whole grain pasta, or a wheat dish. Supplement the staple with one or two colorful vegetables, such as carrots and kale or broccoli and a vegetable salad. Homemade whole wheat bread tastes good without margarine or butter; chapattis or corn tortillas are also good breads. An occasional soy or other bean product will ensure a good source of phytochemicals, along with vitamins, protein, and complex carbohydrates. For a dessert rich in vitamin C, try a sweet piece of fruit. The plant kingdom includes scores of different foods for you to experiment with and learn to enjoy. These foods can be eaten in amounts to make you feel full—not stuffed—and when eaten thus can help you maintain your ideal weight.

Eating a variety of plant-based unrefined whole foods sufficient to maintain weight will automatically ensure sufficient protein. Practically speaking, protein deficiency is impossible except in cases of food shortage. Whole foods also contain the minimum essential fatty acids. Most adults do not need to add any visible fat to their menus. Cereals, legumes, and green leafy vegetables need minimum cooking to break down cellulose envelopes and help make some nutrients more digestible. Follow these simple rules, and you will have little need to worry about individual nutrients.

Many express concern about vitamin B-12, an essential nutrient for the production of red blood cells, nerve sheaths, and DNA. It appears to come entirely as a product of beneficial bacteria. These bacteria are common in all animals; therefore, B-12 is often considered an animal product to be consumed in meat and dairy products. But vitamin B-12 is also produced by normal bacteria in the human mouth and intestine. In addition, it is produced by bacteria in soil and can easily contaminate plant foods or get into ground-water. It is postulated in many poorly sanitated areas that vegetarians obtain sufficient B-12 from unclean vegetables or ground water.[48] Because of the body's ability to store and reuse the vitamin, deficiency often takes 20 or more years to develop. Large amounts of B-12 are stored mainly in the liver. From there, it is excreted in the bile into the bowel and efficiently reabsorbed in the terminal ileum of the small intestine. Deficiencies of vitamin B-12 usually occur in situations in which there is interference with absorption or an imbalance in intake.

Large amounts of vitamins, especially B-1 and C, destroy B-12. Their excessive intake can produce a B-12 deficiency. A high-protein diet also produces a need for more B-12; people on a balanced low-protein diet suffer deficiencies less often than meat eaters. Spirulina and many other products which advertise themselves as a source of B-12 actually contain only B-12 breakdown products and not the vitamin itself. In fact, the breakdown products tend to block the absorption of B-12 and may themselves lead to deficiencies.[49]

Deficiencies of B-12 are most commonly seen as a serious type of anemia (pernicious anemia) or nerve degeneration. Although rare, these must be reckoned with and avoided. Since daily amounts as small as one-tenth of a microgram can cure B-12 deficiencies, large supplements are contraindicated. Such small amounts are needed that deficiency never becomes a problem for most people. (One pound of vitamin B-12 is more than enough to meet the needs of all Americans for an entire year.)[50] If you wonder about sufficient intake, eat soy, cereals, or yeast foods fortified with B-12 or take small supplements of B-12, not more than one microgram per day.

Obviously, if one already has medical problems and/or is taking medications, individual attention to diet and nutrition needs to be received from one's treating physician or a nutritionist. Simple recommendations or minimum requirements do not always hold under such circumstances.

Diet and Spirituality

God says we are to give glory to Him in our eating. This becomes very meaningful when we realize that what we eat can directly affect how clearly we think and understand God and His will for us. The relationship between thinking and diet is stated in the prophecy of the coming Messiah. "Curds and honey He shall eat, that He may know to refuse the evil and choose the good."[51] "Curds and honey" is symbolic language for the best in food and nutrition and is used thus in a number of scriptures. The principle is that one's ability to "know to refuse the evil and choose the good" is dependent on what one eats.

The wise man, Solomon, points out that you are blessed when "your princes feast at the proper time—for strength and not for drunkenness!"[52] Modern medical scientists are beginning to understand that there is a relationship between voluntary restraint and spirituality. Dr. Dean Ornish states,

> I believe that just the act of having voluntary restraints is beneficial to us. When we choose not to eat something when we might otherwise do so, the effect is to make the act of eating more special, more sacred, and thus more joyful. Also, voluntary restraints help us to break free of our compulsions and our addictions . . . *self-imposed* limitations can help to free us. . . . What appears like self-restraint can be self-empowerment. Ultimately, it's a choice between true freedom or being a slave to our compulsions.[53]

Adam and Eve lost their garden home by indulgence of appetite. Diet was important in preparing the children of Israel, under Moses' leadership, for their entry into the Promised Land. Only as we learn, with God's help, to control our appetites can we hope to be ready for Christ's second coming and our heavenly home. We must learn to overcome where Adam and Eve failed.

All people should study practical nutrition for themselves, and a nutrition/cooking school should be established in each church. Observe carefully the effects of what you eat. Feel the difference between good nutrition and bad. Recognize that taste is mostly a learned sensation. If you are willing to make the effort, you can learn to like the delicate flavors of new vegetables and fruits. Accept the challenge of experimentation! Eat to live and don't consider food an end in itself. Food is a requirement for health and clear thinking, but God delights in our enjoyment of the original diet He designed for us. With God's help we can glorify Him in our eating and experience His blessing to us in clearer thinking and greater physical vitality.

---

[1] Revelation 14:6.

[2] 1 Corinthians 10:31.

[3] Davidson, Passmore, Brock, & Truswell, *Human Nutrition and Dietetics* (Churchill Livingstone, 1975) 15.

[4] Sebrell & Haggerty, *Life Science Library—Food and Nutrition* (TIME Inc., 1967).

[5] Ibid, 103-105.

[6] Genesis 1:29.

[7] Genesis 3:17, 18.

[8] Genesis 5.

[9] Genesis 9:3, 4.

[10] Leviticus 3:17.

[11] See Genesis 11.

[12] Temple & Burkitt, *Western Diseases: Their Dietary Prevention and Reversibility* (Human Press, 1994) 129.

[13] Fred Hardinge, "New Findings Challenge Traditional Beliefs," *Adventist Review* 7 Nov. 1991: 20.

[14] Dean Ornish, *Eat More, Weigh Less* (Harper Collins, 1993) 32, 33.

[15] Messina, Messina & Setchell, *The Simple Soybean and Your Health* (Avery, 1994) 154.

[16] McDougall & McDougall, *The McDougall Plan* (New Century Publishers, 1983) 14-17.

[17] Temple & Burkitt, Ibid, 23.

[18] Peter Burwash, *Garuda Indonesia* (Garuda Airline, 1992) 35.

[19] Lester R. Brown, "Facing Food Scarcity," *World Watch* Nov.-Dec. 1995: 11.

[20] Ibid, 12.

[21] Ibid, 13, 14.

[22] Jeremiah 12:11.

[23] Lester R. Brown, Ibid, 15.

[24] Matthew 24:7.

[25] Lester R. Brown, Ibid, 15, 16.

[26] Alan B. Durning, "Fat of the Land," *World Watch* May-June 1991: 12.

[27] Alan B. Durning, "Eating Green," *Nutrition Action Health Letter* Jan.-Feb. 1992: 5.

[28] David & Marcia Pimentel, "Counting the Kilocalories," *CERES* (UN-FAO) Sept.-Oct. 1977: 17-21.

[29] Alan B. Durning, "Fat of the Land," *World Watch* May-June 1991: 13.

[30] Alan B. Durning, "Eating Green," *Nutrition Action Health Letter* Jan.-Feb. 1992: 5.

[31] Alan B. Durning, "Fat of the Land," *World Watch* May-June 1991: 11.

[32] Ibid, 14, 15.

[33] John Robbins, *Diet for a New America* (Stillpoint Publishers, 1987) 365.

[34] Kenneth H. Cooper, MD, *Antioxidant Revolution* (Thomas Nelson Publishers, 1994) 10-12.

[35] Cooper, Ibid, 18-28.

[36] Ibid, 187-189.

[37] Ibid, 38-41.

[38] The daily supplements recommended by Dr. Kenneth Cooper are vitamin E, 200 - 1200 milligrams or international units (IU); beta carotene, 10,000 - 50,000 IU (6 - 30 milligrams); vitamin C, 500 - 3,000 milligrams.

[39] Greenberg, et al, "Mortality Associated with Low Plasma Concentration of Beta Carotene and the Effect of Oral Supplementation," *Journal of the American Medical Association* 6 Mar. 1996: 699-703.

[40] Messina, Messina, & Setchell, Ibid, 16, 17.

[41] Ibid, 71-76.

[42] Ibid, 116-121.

[43] Ibid, 39.

[44] Ibid, 84, 85.

[45] Isaiah 55:2.

[46] Daniel 1:15.

[47] Dean Ornish, MD, *Eat More, Weigh Less* (Harper Perrenial, 1993) 56-58.

[48] Mervyn G. Hardinge, personal conversation, May 1996.

[49] Victor Herbert, "Vitamin B-12," *American Journal of Clinical Nutrition,* Proceedings of the First International Congress on Vegetarian Nutrition, supplement vol. 48, Sept. 1988: 852-858.

[50] Messina, Messina, & Setchell, Ibid, 152, 153.

[51] Isaiah 7:15.

[52] Ecclesiastes 10:17.

[53] Ornish, Ibid, 73, 74.

CHAPTER FIVE

Drink to the Glory of God

DRINK . . . TO THE GLORY OF GOD. 1 CORINTHIANS 10:31

P aul makes it clear we should also drink "to the glory of God."[1] We are still speaking in context of the first angel's message in Revelation 14. We have already recognized that one way to glorify God is by caring for our bodies.[2] One indispensable substance for a healthy body is water.

Drinking Water

The availability of water in liquid form is one of the basic conditions of life on earth and one of God's great gifts. Respiration, digestion, glandular secretion, temperature regulation, sufficient blood volume to maintain circulation, excretion of wastes, and virtually all other body activities depend on water. It acts as a lubricant, helps protect tissues from external injury, and gives flexibility to muscles, tendons, cartilage, and bones. Every chemical and physical function of life is carried out in a water medium.[3]

On average, 57 percent of total body weight in men is water; this equals about 40 liters (42.5 quarts) in a 70-kilogram male. Of this water, about 60 percent is located within body cells, while 40 percent remains fluid outside cells.[4] The water content of a newborn infant is 75 percent of its weight; water balance in a baby is therefore more important than in adults. The volume of body water gradually declines from birth to old age. The amount of water in various tissues varies, with the most active tissues containing the most water. Dry, marrow-free bones are 20 to 25 percent water. Muscles are about 75 percent water, and the gray matter of the brain is 85 percent water.[5] A good brain is mostly water!

The kidneys are vital organs for maintaining a body's water balance and also for serving as the body's main chemical waste disposal system. Ten quarts of blood (about twice the total supply) are filtered through the kidneys every hour; also, the kidneys maintain a close range of salts and electrolytes, glucose, acid-base balance, and other substances in the blood. Waste products are extracted from the blood by the kidneys, and most are expelled in urine. This includes those produced by routine metabolism, in addition to many others that gain entrance through food, beverages, medicines, or by absorption through skin or by inhalation. The heaviest work of the kidney is dealing with urea, the end product of protein metabolism.[6] There is increasing evidence that a prolonged high-protein diet can overwork and damage the kidneys. The higher the protein intake, the greater the work load put on the kidneys and the larger the need for extra water to help flush out the urea.

Ideally the body maintains a balance between the amount of water lost each day and the amount taken in to replace it. Dehydration results in fatigue, which leads to exhaustion, fever, decreased alertness, mental depression, irritability, and coma and death in extreme cases. Thirst is not a sufficient stimulus for drinking enough water. Humans seem to be the only animals that produce in themselves a temporary voluntary dehydration. Unless they force themselves, humans normally replace only about two-thirds of the water they lose when breathing, perspiring heavily, or otherwise losing large amounts of water. People need to make an effort to drink extra water under extreme circumstances.

The following is the daily loss of water (in milliliters) from the average human body:

	Normal Temperature	Hot Weather	Prolonged Heavy Exercise
Insensible loss:			
Skin	350	350	350
Respiratory tract	350	250	650
Urine	1400	1200	500
Sweat	100	1400	5000
Feces	100	100	100
Total	2300	3300	6600[7]

(30 ml = 1 ounce; 8 ounces = 1 cup; 8 cups = 1 quart; 1,000 ml = 1 liter x 1.06 = 1 quart.)

The "insensible loss" through the skin is the invisible perspiration that keeps the skin from drying out and cracking. Visible sweating during hot weather or heavy exercise can be more—as much as 1,500 ml/hour. Insensible loss through the respiratory tract is the unnoticed amount that comes out with each breath. In heavy exercise and in very dry atmospheres, such as on high mountains, this may be a considerable amount. The first successful ascent of Mt. Everest by Hillary and Tenzing is credited to the fact that all climbers on that expedition were urged to force fluids to make up for excessive water loss at such a high altitude.

Up to 10 liters (2-1/2 gallons) of digestive juices are produced daily by the salivary glands, stomach, intestines, liver, and pancreas. The vast majority of the juices are reabsorbed after finishing their work, so only about 100 ml is normally excreted in the feces. This is true except in cases of diarrhea, when massive amounts of fluid are passed from the bowel. This can be deadly, especially in infants, very young children, and the elderly. Even then, it is not the diarrhea that kills, but the dehydration that naturally follows. Oral rehydration therapy (ORT) now saves millions of young children who formerly would have died without this simple treatment.

Water is normally replaced in the body through three sources: (1) water in food, approximately four cups per day; (2) oxidation and metabolism of food, usually one cup each day—more if lots of starchy carbohydrates are eaten; and (3) drinking water, around five cups per day. As pointed out in Chapter 4, it is best to drink water before eating or a couple hours after, but not with meals.

Drinking water even assists in weight control. A person can mistake thirst for hunger. At such times a good drink of cool water can satisfy the body more than eating, and it has no calories. Extra fat in the body requires extra water intake—an extra glass per day for every 25 pounds of excess weight. Also, be aware that salt retains water in the body. Those who eat large amounts of salt need to drink more water to help flush out excess salt, a practice which also reduces weight.[8]

Drinking lots of water not only enables the kidneys to function more effectively, but it is also helps prevent kidney and bladder infections and stone formation. It is almost impossible to initiate either infection or stone formation in diluted urine. Concentrated urine is generally dark yellow. A good indicator of sufficient water intake is if the urine is very pale or clear at least once a day. How much suffering and distress could be relieved if everyone drank sufficient pure water to keep the urine clear.

But there is an increasing problem finding pure, clean water. Although water is our most abundant resource, covering about 71 percent of the earth's surface, 97 percent of it is salt water. Of the remaining 3 percent fresh water, all but 0.003 percent is highly polluted, lies too far under the earth's surface to be affordably extracted, or is locked up in glaciers, polar ice caps, atmosphere, and soil. To put this in measurements we can understand, if the world's water supply were 100 liters (26 gallons), our usable supply of fresh water would be only 0.003 liter (one-half teaspoon).[9] Finding potable water is a growing problem.

Drinking contaminated water is the most common hazard to people in much of the world. Unfortunately, more than 700 contaminants have been found in public drinking water, including (a) organic chemicals like pesticides and solvents, which can cause cancer or harm the nervous system, liver, or kidneys and (b) inorganic chemicals like lead and mercury (which damage the nervous system), nitrates (which cause "blue baby" syndrome), and metals like iron and zinc (which some of us don't get enough of).[10]

The World Bank estimates (1993) that 1.3 billion people in the developing world lack access to clean water, and nearly two billion lack an adequate system for disposing of feces. Without abundant water in or near the home, hygiene becomes difficult or impossible. Lack of water and sanitation is the primary reason that diseases transmitted via feces are so common in developing countries. The most important of these are diarrhea and intestinal worm infections, which account for 10 percent of developing country disease. An inadequate or contaminated water supply also increases the risk of schistosome (bilharzia) infection, skin and eye infections, and guinea worm disease.[11]

Poor water quality is caused by contaminated sources and/or poor distribution systems. Pipes can break or corrode, allowing contamination by sewer lines or other polluted water. Not infrequently, water at its source is clean, but at its point of use is contaminated. Obviously, the point of use at home is the most important place for assuring potable drinking water.

Good sources of drinking water are clean, well-kept, rain collection systems and uncontaminated springs and wells. Recognizing how difficult it is for many people to have access to these, one has to consider water purification or treatment. Simply storing clear water for three days in containers that prevent further contamination gives enough time for most germs to die. The most universally recommended treatment of drinking water is at least five minutes of boiling. In fact, hot water from the tap, if too hot to hold in your hand, provides sufficient heat to kill most bacteria even if it has not been boiled. In many places the problem with having to heat or boil water is the amount of energy required. Most of the world suffers from inadequate and expensive fuel.

Filtration, alone or in combination with activated carbon adsorption, is the most widely used home water treatment. Filters themselves can be hazardous if not kept clean. They can plug up with impurities that can then become a source of contamination. Ultrafiltration and reverse osmosis give the best water available for the lowest price expended.[12]

Chemical treatment with chlorine or iodine preparations is effective, but not practical for everyday home treatment. For personal treatment of small amounts of water, iodine is more effective than chlorine in killing amoebae. The chemicals themselves can be a hazard under certain conditions, but generally are not near the hazard that contaminated water (or not drinking water at all) would be. Municipalities build in safeguards when using chlorine in large water supplies. For certain, there are far fewer chemicals in municipally treated water than in most soft drinks, which contain large amounts of sugar and many other additives.

Average Americans consume more soft drinks than water, another excellent example of spending money for what is not food.[13] The annual (1985) consumption rate per person was soft drinks, 44.5 gallons; water, 44.3 gallons; coffee, 26.3 gallons; beer, 23.8 gallons; milk, 20.1 gallons; and tea, juice, wine, and other alcoholic beverages, 23.5 gallons. Why dilute and contaminate water, one of our most necessary nutrients, with so many chemicals which have no nutrient value beyond sugar and calories? The preference for soft drinks over water is a classic example of perverted appetite.[14]

Soft drinks are mostly a sweet source of water, containing between eight and 12 teaspoons of sugar per 12-ounce serving. Sweet drinks absorb quickly, causing a rapid increase in blood sugar, which then stimulates insulin release. This then stimulates a tendency for blood sugar to fall to a level lower than original, and is a frequent cause of hypoglycemia. Phosphoric acid, present in many soft drinks, tends to deplete body calcium, a definite hazard to those prone to osteoporosis. Why do we upset body balances by taking in unnecessary chemicals?

The caffeine present in cola drinks, coffee, and tea actually has a tendency to dehydrate a person because of its diuretic effect. A person drinking a caffeine beverage should at least drink extra water to make up for the water lost in urine. This is also true of alcoholic beverages.

Whatever its source, drinking water remains a necessity for life. Give your kidneys a treat and help them serve your body more efficiently by giving them an abundant daily supply of pure water.

Recreational Chemicals

The social drink is common in most world societies. Its use has become customary—coffee breaks at work, tea parties at home, champagne for celebration, toasts (with alcoholic drinks) "to your health." People like these beverages because they make one "feel good"—either more relaxed or more stimulated. Many people use alcoholic drinks excessively because they have become psychologically or chemically dependent on them. Alcoholic drinks are psychotropic (psychoactive) drugs, meaning one of their major effects is an influence on the mind, usually by affecting the neurotransmitters (the chemicals that control the liquid connection between nerve endings).

There are more than 1,500 compounds classified primarily as psychotropic agents. These alter the function of the central nervous system (CNS) as to warrant the designation *psychotoxic*. They include sedatives, tranquilizers, antihypertensives and antidepressants, and neuroleptic drugs. They also include many natural products, such as alcohol, coffee, tea, tobacco, marijuana, LSD, opioids and cocaine, steroids, and cardiac glycosides.[15]

We divide the most commonly used psychotropic substances into two broad categories, stimulants and depressants, depending on their effects in the central nervous system. They provide no nutrients except calories in alcohol and the nutrients that may be added to caffeine beverages in sugar and cream. Their effect is a chemical "drug" effect.

Substances containing caffeine. Common substances containing caffeine include coffee, tea, cola drinks, and chocolate. The amounts of caffeine are assumed by most studies to be 137 mg per cup of coffee, 47 mg per cup of tea, 46 mg per can or bottle of cola beverage, and 7 mg per serving (1 oz) of chocolate candy.[16] This obviously varies according to the strength or concentration of the preparation. The popularity of coffee is seen in the fact that worldwide consumption equals about 10 billion pounds a year.[17]

Caffeine induces a mild euphoria, an increased sense of alertness, and an apparent decrease in fatigue. Inability to sleep and restlessness often accompany caffeine intake. While giving one a temporary "lift," a chemical stimulus is always followed by a depression greater than one had before the "lift." In other words, caffeine has no effect on the fatigue mechanism and is actually causing the mind to believe a lie. When the stimulus is finished, the fatigue and depression can be severe, naturally calling for more of the stimulant. The action is similar to whipping a tired horse. When chemically stimulated, the body will borrow from its reserves and "feel" less tired for a time. But in the long term, the body is stressed, and the immune, central nervous, and cardio-vascular systems suffer.

The illusion of alertness is unmasked when tested by performance. A person under the influence of caffeine is able to type faster, but will make more errors. Judgment is influenced in that a person will think he is doing better he actually is. Reaction time and reflex responses temporarily improve, but quickly decline to a lower level than when fatigue was first noted. The letdown and decreased efficiency when caffeine wears off is frequently interpreted as a demand for more caffeine. (This is how the process of addiction gets started. The body can quickly become habituated and chemically dependent so that a person cannot perform normally without the chemical being present. Without the chemical, withdrawal symptoms such as headache, tremor, and nervousness occur.)

In addition to influencing the mind, caffeine can also predispose the heart to irregular beat—premature beats and fast rate. Blood flow to most of the body is increased, but circulation to the brain is decreased. The stomach and gastrointestinal system are directly stimulated by the oils in coffee, sometimes leading to diarrhea. This stomach irritation, incidentally, is even greater with decaffeinated coffee than with regular.[18]

Why do people "spend money for what is not bread and your wages for what does not satisfy? . . . eat [and drink] what is good, and let your soul delight itself in abundance."[19]

Alcohol. "Alcohol has the unique distinction of being the only potent pharmacological agent with which obvious self-induced intoxication is socially acceptable."[20] As a drug, alcohol is readily absorbed directly from the stomach and duodenum and can be found almost immediately in the blood, which carries it to all the body. It tends to concentrate in the body's organs in proportion to their water content. Its toxic effects are primarily noted in the brain and liver. It actually functions in the CNS as an anesthetic, putting one to sleep and killing some of the brain cells, especially in the frontal lobe where judgment, self-control, psychologic inhibitions, and conscience are located. The depression of normal inhibitions causes many people to loosen up and become boisterous. This is not stimulation but depression of the ability to think clearly.

Poor reaction time and loss of nervous reflexes and judgment lead to around 100,000 deaths each year in the U.S. Nearly half of all accidental deaths, suicides, and murders are alcohol-related. The ninth most common cause of death in the U.S. is alcoholic cirrhosis. Much of the cell damage that occurs during liver degeneration is believed to be caused by free radicals liberated during alcohol metabolism.[21] Alcohol is a common cause of malnutrition, high blood pressure, heart disease, and cancer—especially of the stomach, liver, lung, pancreas, colon, and tongue. It suppresses the bone marrow's capacity to produce white blood cells and thus seriously interferes with the immune system. Drinking during pregnancy is one of the top three causes of birth defects in the U.S., causing stunted growth, mental retardation, malformed facial features, and lifelong heart problems. Alcohol rivals tobacco in being the most widely used and destructive drug.[22]

Alcohol is used in several forms. The oldest and only form of alcoholic drink in Bible times was fermented wine or beer. Distillation was not developed until around A.D. 500. Whatever its form, a "drink" is 1.5 ounces of whiskey, gin, or other distilled spirit; 5 ounces of wine; or a 12-ounce can of beer—each of which contains about the same amount of alcohol. Most Biblical counsel about alcohol seems to be consistent with this theme: "Wine is a mocker, strong drink is a brawler, and whoever is led astray by it is not wise."[23]

Approximately 75 percent of Americans drink alcohol, and one in 10 experience problems with alcoholism.[24] It is impossible, however, to accurately predict who will be the one drinker in ten to experience problems. Alcoholism is the physical dependency on continued use of alcohol, in which bodily damage occurs as listed above, or a person becomes tolerant (addicted) to the substance and cannot stop drinking without serious physical effects such as tremor, weakness, sweating, hyperreflexia, and GI symptoms. In severe withdrawal, grand mal seizures and hallucinations, confusion, poor sleep, and frightening dreams (delirium tremens) occur.

Alcohol abuse deprives men and women of the superlatives in life. Enjoyment is blurred or absent in areas of real living—such as recreation, music, art, eating, sex, and conversation. Some people hesitate to walk with Christ because they do not want to give up certain "pleasures," but God promises, "No good thing will He withhold from them that walk uprightly."[25] They need to understand that biblical regulations were written so that man might obtain the greatest amount of joy from life.[26]

Other Psychotropic Substances. Since there are more than 1,500 known psychotropic drugs, we limit this discussion to those which are most abused and commonly cause dependence. Drug abuse is defined in terms of societal disapproval and involves different type of behavior: (1) experimental and recreational use of illegal (unprescribed) drugs; (2) unwarranted use of psychoactive drugs to relieve problems or symptoms; and (3) use of drugs at first for the above reasons, with later development of dependence and continuation to avoid the discomfort of withdrawal.

Drugs that produce dependence act on the central nervous system to produce one or more of the following effects: reduced anxiety and tension, elation and euphoria (pleasurable feelings), feelings of increased mental and physical ability, altered sensory perception, and changes in behavior. These drugs include (1) CNS depressants which, other than alcohol, include opioid pain relievers such as morphine, codeine, and demerol; and the barbiturates and other sedatives; (2) tranquilizers such as Valium (diazepam), Librium, and Xanax; (3) CNS stimulants, including caffeine, amphetamines ("speed"), and cocaine; and (4) hallucinogens such as marijuana, mescaline, peyote, and LSD.[27]

These affect the mind by distorting its ability to relate to reality and causing it to "believe a lie."[28] Their influence makes it impossible to know the truth and discriminate between right and wrong; judgment is perverted and behavior is often not rational. For these reasons, in addition to their many adverse effects on body systems, all psychotropic substances should be avoided except in rare cases where needed for pain relief or to medically treat severe agitation.

Healing Water

Water internally is necessary for life, and externally it can be a powerful medicine. Regular, preferably daily, cleansing with soap and water maintains healthy skin. Someone has figured that the average person has more living organisms threatening infection on his skin than the world has human inhabitants.[29] However, too much hot water with soap eliminates the protective oils in the skin, leads to dryness and itching, and can thus increase the potential for infections.

Water possesses physical and chemical properties that make it an ideal agent for transferring hot and cold to the body. Its very abundance, availability, economy, and ease of use make it one of the blessings of heaven for application as a simple and rational remedy. It is the universal solvent, non-irritating, and its viscosity is perfect for easy use.[30] Within a comparatively limited range of temperature, water exists in three different states: solid ice, liquid, and gaseous vapor. This makes it comparatively simple to use the different states as treatment.

The body responds dramatically to heat and cold. The **intrinsic** effects of cold are seen in a body which has been long exposed to either cold air or water. If thoroughly chilled, body functions are slowed or depressed. The respiration, pulse, and circulation slow; skin sensation is blunted; muscles move sluggishly and clumsily; digestion is arrested; and body temperature lowers. While cold depresses, the intrinsic effects of moderate heat stimulate life processes. Respiration, pulse, and circulation increase; digestion proceeds more rapidly; muscles are more quick and active; and skin sensations are more quickly perceived.

However, if heat or cold are applied briefly, the body experiences the opposite of the intrinsic effects. For instance, when cold is applied briefly to a warm body, the **reactionary** effect is for the heart to beat more rapidly and forcibly; the circulation is whipped up; the nerves tingle with new life; respiration becomes at first rapid, then slower and deeper; and the muscles are energized. It is as if the body, anticipating the intrinsic depressing effect of cold, counteracts by increasing the vigor of the vital processes. The reaction effect is thus the opposite of the intrinsic effect. Therefore, the reaction to heat is recognized as depression of body functions. Many of the most beneficial results of hydrotherapy are due to reaction effects, not the intrinsic effects of heat and cold. Incidentally, reactions do not occur well in the very young or old or in those who are greatly weakened. The body must have good vital force to produce reactionary effects.

Reactions include different phases. A **thermic reaction** to cold causes the body to produce more heat. The skin becomes reddened due to increased circulation, the **circulatory reaction**. The nerves tingle as with new life, the **nervous reaction**. The phase most apparent is the circulatory reaction, so the skin color is an excellent indicator of the completeness of a reaction.[31]

The benefits of hydrotherapy include the following:

- it arouses the body to bring about its own recuperation and healing. This is increasingly important in treating infections as antibiotics face the problem of drug resistance. A recent *Journal of the American Medical Association* recognizes this problem when it states,

  > Unfortunately, the increasing widespread emergence of acquired resistance to antibiotics over the last 40 years now constitutes a serious threat to global public health. . . . Bacterial resistance has rendered useless a number of previously valuable antibiotic treatments and now threatens the effectiveness of others.[32]

- it provides natural tonic (stimulating) or sedative effects which do not have the common aftereffects of drugs.

Because the body works hard to distribute heat and cold, local applications do not directly penetrate deep organs. There is abundant evidence, however, that applications to the skin do have strong effects on deep or distant organs. This is accounted for by the reflex effects that are mediated by nerves to the central nervous system and which affect the circulatory system. Generally, the reflex or distant effects are the same as the local skin effects.

It is generally true that every organ is in reflex relation to the skin immediately over it. In some instances, however, the skin in one area has a strong reflex influence on distant internal organs. For instance, the following local applications produce distant reflex effects:[33]

Local Skin Applications	Distant Organs Affected (reflexively)
The face, scalp, and back of neck	Brain
The neck	Pharynx and larynx
The back of the neck	Mucus membranes of the nose
The chest and shoulders	Lungs
Lower right chest	Liver
Lower left chest	Spleen
Lower third of sternum	Kidneys
Lower dorsal and lumbar spine	Kidneys and intestines
Lower lumbar and sacral spine	Pelvic organs
Epigastrium	Stomach
Feet and legs	Brain, lungs, and pelvic organs
Hands	Brain and nasal mucus membrane

Although simple, hydrotherapy is a science to be learned from those experienced in it. Here are a few examples of applications of hydrotherapy:

- Prolonged immersion of hands in cold water causes contraction of the blood vessels of the nasal mucus membranes.
- Short, cold applications to the face and head stimulate mental activity.
- An ice bag applied over the heart slows the heart rate, increases its force, and raises arterial blood pressure.
- A short, cold application such as a cold rub to the chest at first increases respiration but soon results in deeper breathing with a slowed rate.
- A prolonged heat application to any area of skin reflexly produces dilation of the blood vessels in the distant organ.
- Hot, moist applications (fomentations) to the chest facilitate respiration and expectoration.
- Prolonged, hot applications to the abdomen lessen peristalsis (and colic).

The short (one minute) cold application has been said to be more useful and desirable in changing the functions of the body than any other form of therapeutics. In addition to circulatory effects, the skin is toned, basal metabolism increases, red and white blood cells increase, urine production increases, and constipation is relieved. Heat applications usually bring more blood to an area, stimulate the work of white blood cells in fighting infection, and can relax muscles and relieve muscle spasm pain.

Alternate hot and cold applications can promote the best of both. This is done by placing the part in hot water (105-110 degrees Fahrenheit) for three or four minutes, followed by cold water (preferably ice water) for 30 to 60 seconds. This should be repeated six to eight times, beginning with hot and ending with cold. By alternately contracting and dilating blood vessels, it produces "vascular exercise," markedly increasing blood flow to the treated area (and its reflex organ) and thus hastening healing. It also increases phagocytic and immunity responses, increasing both the number and activity of white blood cells. This helps treat infection. Alternate hot and cold also tends to reduce swelling and decrease pain in the treated area. It can truly be powerful medicine for many infections, and it hastens healing of most injuries.[34]

Another simple, effective treatment is warm vapor inhalation for upper respiratory infections such as colds. This can relieve inflammation and congestion of the upper respiratory mucus membrane, relieve throat irritation, loosen secretions, and relieve coughing. It is done by heating water to boiling in a kettle and then placing a towel over the head in such a way as to catch the steam. Take care not to burn the patient or set fire to bedding or clothing. Have the patient breathe the water vapor slowly and deeply for 30 minutes to an hour. Repeat two or three times per day. A little eucalyptus or pine oil in the water helps give the desire to inhale, but hot air is the treating force. Patients treated this way will seldom need to go to a doctor for treatment of common respiratory infections.[35]

Other home treatments include massage for its mechanical and reflex circulatory effects; the internal and external use of charcoal for its poison adsorbing and healing effects; and the use of some medicinal herbs, such as garlic internally or aloe vera externally. All treatments have precautions to follow, but the simple treatments mentioned here are comparatively harmless and work effectively in many situations.

All are encouraged to learn simple home remedies for treating the majority of illnesses. If improvement is not quickly seen, however, the sick person should be promptly taken to a doctor or hospital for their advice. Never continue to treat patients at home whose condition is getting worse. This is particularly true for infants and small children. With these precautions, rest assured that God blesses use of water and His natural resources for home treatment of sickness. Churches should recognize themselves as simple health centers, and classes in home treatments such as hydrotherapy should be given both to members and to the community. This kind of medical missionary work is referred to in Chapter 9.

Spiritual Summary

Life as we know it cannot exist without water, one of the most useful and necessary substances on earth. Essentially all body functions, both physical and chemical, require water. It cleanses, refreshes, and is vital for plant growth. Water can be a powerful aid in helping the body restore its function.

It is expected that anything so good would counterfeited and contaminated by the devil. Certainly this is true with water. Many have come to prefer soft drinks and other adulterated beverages to pure water. In some places, potable water is not available due to the contaminated environment. The devil's master deception is to control or interfere with our minds through the promotion and popularity of alcoholic drinks and other psychoactive substances.

Through Jeremiah, God counseled,

For My people have committed two evils: they have forsaken Me, the fountain of living waters, and hewn themselves cisterns, broken cisterns that can hold no water.[36]

Our efforts to be independent of God are like broken cisterns that cannot hold water. Eternal life is dependent on our acceptance of God's gift of spiritual water. Jesus said to the Samaritan woman,

Whoever drinks of this (well) water will thirst again, but whoever drinks of the water that I shall give him will never thirst. But the water that I shall give him will become in him a fountain of water, springing up into everlasting life.[37]

That we receive this spiritual water (the Holy Spirit) to bless others is amplified in these words of Jesus:

If anyone thirsts, let him come to Me and drink. He who believes in Me, as the Scripture has said, out of his heart will flow rivers of living water.[38]

Some of God's final words in the Bible are this beautiful invitation: "'Come!' And let him who thirsts come. Whoever desires, let him take the water of life freely."[39] God seeks to satisfy us with good things, but we must desire and choose His way in proper use of water as one step in receiving His gifts. By helping the body function more efficiently and by preventing intoxication and irrational thinking, we will glorify God as the first angel commanded.

---

[1] 1 Corinthians 10:31.
[2] 1 Corinthians 6:19, 20.
[3] Mervyn G. Hardinge, *A Philosophy of Health* (School of Health, 1980) 37.
[4] Arthur C. Guyton, *Human Physiology and Mechanisms of Disease,* 4th ed. (W. B. Saunders Co., 1987) 267, 268.
[5] Hardinge, Ibid, 37.
[6] J. D. Ratcliff, *I Am Joe's Body* (The Reader's Digest, 1975) 159-164.
[7] Guyton, Ibid, 267.
[8] Vernon W. Foster, MD, *NEWSTART* (Woodbridge Press, 1988) 95.

[9] G. Tyler Miller, Jr., *Living in the Environment* (Wadsworth Publishing, 1990) 238.

[10] "Water: Treat it Right," *Nutrition Action Healthletter* Nov. 1990: 5.

[11] World Bank, *World Development Report 1993* (Oxford University Press, 1993) 90, 91.

[12] John Schaeffer, *Alternative Energy Sourcebook,* 7th ed. (Real Goods Trading Corp., 1993) 81-87.

[13] Isaiah 55:2.

[14] Myron Winick, MD, "Soft Drink Alert," *The Book of Inside Information* (New York: Boardroom Classics, 1989) 441.

[15] Gilman, Goodwin & Gilman, "Drugs and the Treatment of Psychiatric Disorders," *The Pharmacological Basis of Therapeutics,* 6th ed. (Macmillan Publishing, 1980) 391.

[16] Walter C. Willett, et al, "Coffee Consumption and Coronary Heart Disease in Women," *Journal of the American Medical Association* 14 Feb. 1996: 459.

[17] Vernon W. Foster, MD, Ibid, 130.

[18] Gilman, Goodman & Gilman, Ibid, 604.

[19] Isaiah 55:2.

[20] Gilman, Goodman & Gilman, Ibid, 551.

[21] "Alcohol and the Liver," *Alcohol Alert,* National Institute on Alcohol Abuse and Alcoholism, Jan. 1993: 2.

[22] Tufts University *Diet & Nutrition Letter,* vol. 7, no. 10, Dec. 1989: 3-5.

[23] Proverbs 20:1.

[24] Robert Berkow, MD, ed., "Dependence on Alcohol," *Merck Manual,* 16th ed. (1992) 1552.

[25] Psalm 84:11, KJV.

[26] S. I. McMillen, MD, "Robber of Ten Million Brains," *None of These Diseases* (Fleming H. Revell, 1984) 32.

[27] Robert Berkow, MD, ed., "Drug Dependence," *Merck Manual,* 16th ed., 1992: 1549, 1550.

[28] 2 Thessalonians 2:11.

[29] Vernon W. Foster, MD, Ibid, 37.

[30] Agatha and Calvin Thrash, *Home Remedies* (Thrash Publications, 1981) 51-53.

[31] Charles S. Thomas, Faculty Sponsor, *Water Seminar Syllabus* (LLU School of Health, 1981) 100:12, 13.

[32] Chopra, Hodgson, Metcalf, and Poste, "New Approaches to the Control of Infections Caused by Antibiotic-Resistant Bacteria, An Industry Perspective," *Journal of the American Medical Association* 7 Feb. 1996: 401.

[33] Charles S. Thomas, Adapted from Ibid, 100:20, 21.

[34] Thrash & Thrash, Ibid, 72.

[35] Charles Thomas, *Simple Water Treatments for the Home* (Loma Linda University Press, 1977) 38-43.

[36] Jeremiah 2:11.

[37] John 4:13, 14.

[38] John 7:37, 38.

[39] Revelation 22:17.

CHAPTER SIX

All to the Glory of God

WHATEVER YOU DO, DO ALL TO THE GLORY OF GOD. 1 CORINTHIANS 10:31

The first angel of Revelation 14 says, "Fear God and give glory to Him."[1] Paul points out that "whether you eat or drink, or whatever you do, do all to the glory of God."[2] Our entire lifestyle should point to a good God who is the Creator, Restorer, and Sustainer of His human children. Humans simply cooperate with God and with His help seek to keep the laws of health that are inherent in human anatomy and physiology. The devil, of course, points to the difficulty of living healthily and creates in us desires and passions that are unholy.

In this chapter we look at some important elements of a godly lifestyle.

Physical Fitness

A basic law of our being is "Use it or lose it." Without exercise a person soon loses strength. Physical fitness, the ability of the body to respond to work or stress, is one of the best measures a person's health. The pulse rate after a measured amount of exercise helps determine level of fitness. The higher the pulse after exercise, usually the less fit the person. The treadmill exercise electrocardiogram (EKG) is the technique used by most physicians. Other simple methods include the Kasch Step Test[3] or Cooper's measurement of the distance covered in 12 minutes or the time taken to walk/run 1.5 miles.[4]

The average American male has a resting heart rate (RHR) of about 70 beats per minute; the average American woman, about 75 to 80 beats per minute. (The RHR is ideally taken in the morning just after awakening and before getting up.) Highly trained athletes commonly have RHRs in the mid-40s or lower. All should seek to develop RHRs below 60. Recognize, however, that heart rate tends to slow down with age; some elderly persons may have a low RHR but not be fit.

A lower RHR is usually evidence not only that the person is more fit, but also that the cardiovascular system is more efficient (pumps more blood with less work). In a well-exercised person the heart actually grows stronger, and the number and size of blood vessels and total blood volume increase, thus enabling the body tissues to be more easily saturated with energy-producing oxygen. Even the efficiency of the lungs is increased as they become conditioned to process more air with less effort. Unwanted fat tends to burn up and flabby tissues become strong and firm, making one look and feel better. As physical deterioration and the aging process slow down, one's zest for life and youthful vigor return. It is easier to relax, tolerate stress, and get more work done with less fatigue.

Fit individuals not only have lower RHR, but their heart rates tend to rise more slowly when anxiety strikes or their activity level increases. They are less likely to have serious heart difficulty when suddenly put under pressure or stressed. Coronary heart disease risk is further decreased because exercise increases the good HDL cholesterol, while total cholesterol and triglycerides decrease. As RHR decreases, total blood pressure usually decreases. An optimum fitness level also directly stimulates the production and function of the body's natural antioxidants, which fight damaging free radicals.

Other benefits of physical fitness include these:[5]

- More personal energy
- Less depression, less hypochondria, and less "free-floating" anxiety
- More efficient digestion with less constipation
- Bones increase in strength
- A better self-image and more self-confidence
- Easier pregnancy and childbirth
- More restful sleep
- Fewer aches and pains, including back pain

Exercise—the Body in Motion

The benefits of physical fitness are clear. How does one become fit? Quite simply, by keeping active. Paul was obviously acquainted with the principles of physical training. He advises, "Let us run with endurance [patience] the race that is set before us,"[6] and further challenges, "Run in such a way that you may obtain it (the prize)."[7] The knowledge that one must patiently train in order to win has been with us a long time. The shame is that so few take it seriously. Less than 20 percent (perhaps only 10 percent) of Americans have good exercise programs, half have no exercise habits at all, and the rest have less exercise than is recommended for health.[8]

There are three general types of exercise: (1) **aerobic** or endurance exercise, (2) **flexibility** exercises, and (3) **strength-building** exercises, such as calisthenics and weight-lifting. All are needed, but because of its positive effects on the total cardiovascular-pulmonary system, as well as its general effect on the whole body, aerobic exercise is the most highly recommended. "Aerobics refers to a variety of exercises that stimulate heart and lung activity for a time period sufficiently long to produce beneficial changes in the body."[9] The variety includes running, swimming, jogging, walking, cycling, cross-country skiing, and many others that are of sufficient endurance and intensity to provide a training effect.

The more exercise is studied, the more evident it is that low-intensity exercise, such as walking, is more desirable than high-intensity exercise, such as jogging or running. Intense training is not only accompanied by more accidents and injuries, but studies show that intense training can actually injure the immune system by producing excess free radicals and can be one cause for people being more susceptible to infections.[10] While it may take a little more time, walking can provide all the health benefits of more intense exercise, with much less risk of injury.

Ideally, follow the FIT routine:

Frequency—daily is best, but three to five days per week is a good schedule.

Intensity—60 percent to 80 percent of predicted maximum heart rate (MHR). Calculate MHR by subtracting age from 220 and multiplying by 60 percent and 80 percent. For example, if age is 60: 220 - 60 = 160. 160 x 60% = 96. 160 x 80% = 128. The recommended intensity for this person is to keep the heart rate between 96 and 128 beats per minute.

Time—20 minutes minimum for jogging; 40 minutes for walking. Begin slowly, taking 20 minutes to walk a mile, and gradually increase over six months as fitness improves and heart rate slows until one is able to walk a mile in 12 minutes. Longer periods are ideal, but shorter periods can accumulate benefit. In other words, if 40 minutes is not available in one block of time, lesser amounts can be added together and provide benefit.

Any individual who has been very sedentary or has any indication of heart problems should obtain clearance from a physician before beginning any exercise program. If you cannot follow an ideal schedule, be assured that any exercise is better than none. Always walk up stairs instead of riding the elevator. Seek opportunities to walk instead of drive. Be conscious that to gain or maintain fitness you must keep active. Rejoice at every opportunity you find to exercise. Do useful outside work such as gardening. Ideal exercise provides the satisfaction of doing useful work while you develop fitness.

Next in importance to aerobic exercise is a flexibility/stretching routine. Unused muscles become tight, restrict joint movement, cause pain with an increased potential for injury, and affect posture and body alignment. It is important every day to make sure all joints are put through their full range of motion. This can be done by stretching to the point of comfortable tension and holding that position for five to eight seconds. Never stretch to the point of pain and do not bounce while your muscles are fully stretched. Slowly release tension and repeat eight to ten times. The key to flexibility is frequency and consistency. Proper breathing is also important. Inhale before the stretch and exhale while holding it. You cannot stretch too often, if done correctly. Ideally, all aerobic exercise begins and ends with stretching exercises for five to ten minutes as part of warm-up and cool-down. This is less important for walking exercise.

The third type of exercise—strength building—combines well with both aerobic and flexibility training. If the ideal routine for aerobic exercise is followed and the recommended heart rate is maintained for at least 20 minutes, strength is being built. Calisthenics, which require no equipment and can be done almost anywhere, are also recommended. Strengthening comes by adding repetitions or making routines slightly harder, being careful not to produce injury or become exhausted. Machine or weight exercises have the advantage of enabling you to easily, precisely, and gradually increase your strength. To avoid injury, always begin with a weight that you are certain is too light and work up gradually to heavier weights. A good routine is to begin with the large muscles of the legs, then work with the middle and upper back, chest, shoulders, arms, and abdominal muscles.

Nothing produces the feeling of vibrant health more than regular exercise and staying fit. Not only does a physically fit person cut his heart attack risk in half, but he also slows the aging process. But it is not the physiological benefits that motivate most people; the psychological benefits of feeling well are probably more important. Exercise stimulates the secretion of endorphins from the pituitary gland. These have a morphine-like action which helps produce a natural euphoria and can help control pain. Many psychiatrists prescribe exercise as treatment for mental depression.

Perhaps the most beneficial use of exercise for mental health, however, is as a natural tranquilizer. Nothing works better to reduce anxiety and nervous tension than a good physical workout. Overstimulation of the nervous system, so common in times of stress, produces catecholamines which are poison to the body, especially the heart.[11] These harmful products of adrenaline stimulation can only be used up or neutralized by physical exercise. The body is clearly designed so that nervous tension should be balanced with physical exercise. Because of its tranquilizing effect, moderate exercise an hour or two before going to bed can greatly assist the production of restful sleep.

Fresh Air, the Breath of Life

"And the Lord God formed man of the dust of the ground, and breathed into his nostrils the breath of life; and man became a living being."[12] From the eagerly awaited first cry of the newborn to the last gasp of the dying, life is completely dependent on breathing in adequate oxygen and breathing out carbon dioxide. The most important rule of first aid is to assure the airway is open and that breathing or respiration can be maintained. Brain damage begins to occur within about four minutes if breathing stops.

Respiration consists of taking air (which at sea level is about 20 percent oxygen) into the lungs and breathing out carbon dioxide. The respiratory tract includes the nose, nasopharynx, larynx, trachea, bronchi, and the bronchioles, which lead to the more than 300 million air sacs (alveoli) from which the oxygen actually passes into the blood. In the environment, green plants breathe carbon dioxide into tiny pores on the underside of their leaves and breathe out the oxygen required by humans and animals. Nature thus provides the external respiratory cycle.

Internal respiration is the passage of the oxygen from the lungs into the blood, which carries it, largely by red blood cells, to every cell of the body. Within the cells it is the organelles called mitochondria that "burn" fuel (food) in the presence of oxygen to produce the energy required by all cell functions. This metabolism of energy produces carbon dioxide and water. The water is used in the body, but the carbon dioxide is expelled by the cells and quickly picked up by the blood and transported back to the lungs, which breath it out.

The principle muscle of respiration is the diaphragm, a large, flat muscle separating the abdominal from the chest cavity. It acts somewhat like a piston. A good deep breath requires the abdomen to expand to pull down the diaphragm, thus increasing chest capacity. Expiration is largely the passive relaxation of the abdominal muscles and diaphragm. Observation of babies confirms that abdominal breathing is natural, but many people so seldom breathe deeply that they forget how to use the abdomen. Wearing anything tight around the waist prevents deep breathing. Exercise forces deep breathing and increased respiration.

While deep breathing relaxes and reduces stress, it is even more vital for its cleansing, infection-reducing effects. Quiet breathing passes in and out about 500 ml (approximately one pint) of air with each breath. The vital capacity—the total amount that can be passed in and out of the lungs in one breath—is about 4,000 ml, or eight times greater. Inevitably germs get breathed in and can wander easily into the large, seldomly used areas of the lungs. Germs like nothing better than dark, warm, damp areas where they can multiply undisturbed. Deep breathing several times a day is needed to wash out the lungs and help prevent many respiratory infections.

For the world as a whole, acute respiratory disease is the most common cause of death, especially for those under two years old. Respiratory infections are commonly caused by viruses, bacteria, and fungi (molds). Unfortunately, there are also many other hazards to respiration. Long-term inhalation of various dusts into the lungs can lead to scarring and fibrosis of the lungs, which can greatly interfere with breathing. Such dusts are particularly hazardous in mining and some other industries. Since there is no effective treatment, prevention by wearing masks or other protective devices is essential. Other problems come from breathing substances to which a person is allergic. Hay fever and asthma are common mani-festations of allergy.

A particularly large hazard today is the breathing in of gases and other substances in polluted air. During a day in a city, one can inhale up to 17,000 pints of air containing some 20 billion particles of foreign material—dirt, dust, and chem-icals.[13] City air is polluted by carbon monoxide and hydrocarbons (mostly from automobiles), sulfur oxides (from burning coal and fuel oil), particulate matter (particles of solid or liquid matter from industrial processes), nitrogen oxides (from automobiles and steam power plants), and photochemical oxidants. Smog is formed from such substances as ozone—produced by the action of sunlight on hydrocarbons—and nitrogen oxides. All of these can be harmful to health.[14]

The most important air hazard to health is tobacco smoking. Not only does smoking directly damage the lungs of the one smoking, but most of the smoke from a cigarette is sidestream smoke that goes into the atmosphere and harms to those in close contact with smokers. Smoking is the largest single cause of preventable disease in the world today. It causes not only chronic bronchitis, emphysema, and lung cancer and makes one more susceptible to all respiratory infections, but it also causes up to one-third of all heart disease, the most common cause of adult deaths in the Western world. Unfortunately, people in the devel-oping world are increasing their smoking just as the U.S. and some other Western countries are successfully reducing their smoking habits. A major influence is the desire of the tobacco industry to make money off this killer habit.

Air is so essential to life that the body has several defenses for protecting the lungs. First, the hairs in the nose trap the largest air particles. Next the air comes in contact with linings in the nose, which warm and moisten it. Very cold or very dry air can harm the lungs. In the back of the nose and throat, the air comes in contact with the adenoids and tonsils, immune system organs which identify and begin the process of destroying viruses and germs. The respiratory tract lining also contains many mucus-producing cells. Mucus is designed to trap foreign objects and, with the help of active fine hair (cilia) cells, to carry them back up the respiratory tract. The large tubes of the respiratory tract are lined with ciliated cells that constantly move dust and other particles out of the lungs. An early effect of smoking is the paralyza-tion and death of these vital cilia cells. With their loss, the best defense left is coughing or sneezing. Coughing produces a rush of air approaching a speed of 600 miles per hour in its effort to propel debris and mucus up and out of the respiratory tract.[15]

Poor ventilation allows the multiplication and concentration of germs, which leads to increased disease in those who live or work in crowded, poorly ventilated buildings. It is vital that we always have clean, fresh air to breathe. It is also important that we clear out our lungs and give ourselves a good boost of oxygen with frequent deep breathing.

The brain and its nerve cells are the most sensitive in the body to lack of oxygen. A nerve cell will die within four seconds if deprived of oxygen. Fortunately sufficient oxygen is present within the blood and tissues that cells do not immediately lose contact with oxygen when breathing ceases. Because the brain is enclosed in the non-expandable skull, it cannot increase its blood supply the way muscles and other organs do—by expanding blood vessels. There's little room in the skull for expansion. The brain primarily increases it's blood supply (and oxygen) by increasing the body's general circulation. This is best done by exercise.

The Greeks, who walked while discussing topics of importance, were believers in the ability of exercise to improve mental function. . . . Aristotle started his peripatetic (moving about or walking) school in 335 BC. His school was so named because of his habit of walking up and down the paths of the Lyceum in Athens while thinking or lecturing to his students who walked with him. Plato and Socrates also practiced the art of peripatetics.[16]

Christ, of course, did much of His teaching while walking with His disciples. Modern studies suggest that short-term memory, comprehension, and ability to react mentally are all improved by exercise and its stimulation of increased oxygen flow to the brain.[17]

As we recognize the relationship between adequate oxygen intake and mental abilities, breathing becomes even more important to the Christian who seeks to keep his mental powers as sharp as possible. We must give careful thought to how our bodies can best get a good supply of fresh air and prevent common respiratory infections. God has supplied us with an abundance of oxygen-carrying air; we must keep it free of pollution and assume responsibility for how we use it.

Sunshine, the Energy Source

The sun, created by God, is the source of all energy on earth. Life here cannot exist without sunlight. Solar energy (electromagnetic energy from the sun) shines down on earth, where it produces light and heat and is used by plants to photosynthesize chemical energy (food and oxygen). Coal and oil are chemical energy from fossil plants. Chemical energy from plants (fruits, grains, vegetables, etc.) is taken into the body as food directly, or secondhand through animals who ate plants. Food is transformed by digestion and metabolism into work energy for muscle movement, production energy for making enzymes and hormones, and electrical energy for nerve cells and all other body activities. Heat is produced to maintain warmth in the body. Except for atomic energy and God's creation of the world, we normally think of energy as being transferred from one state to another—neither created nor destroyed.

The fact that light was the first thing created during creation week is evidence of its environmental importance. Its benefits are so clear that one can understand why so many throughout history have worshiped the sun.

Light is of three principal types: ultraviolet (UV)—short waves (5 percent); visible light (40 percent); and infrared—long waves (54 percent). The remaining one percent is made up of cosmic rays, gamma rays, x-rays, radio waves, and electric waves. Sunlight helps purify the environment by killing germs. Most bacteria are killed by two hours of exposure to the sun's UV rays; this is true even through most window glass. UV is also responsible for the production of vitamin D in the skin. Vitamin D is needed in calcium metabolism and bone production. In fair-skinned people living in temperate climates, an exposure of the hands and face to fifteen minutes of sun on clear days two or three times a week is sufficient; dark-skinned people require more exposure for the same amount of vitamin D production. As skin grows thinner in old age, the amount of vitamin D produced is less.

Sunshine has been shown to make neutrophils more efficient at ingesting germs and to increase the number of lymphocytes in circulation, thus strengthening the immune system. It tends to normalize blood pressure and decrease blood cholesterol. In diabetics, sunlight lowers blood sugar, apparently by stimulating the beta cells of the pancreas to more efficient production of insulin and by stimulating production of an enzyme, glycogen synthetase, which helps the liver remove glucose from the blood and store it as glycogen. Psychologically, sunshine is a mood elevator, probably by stimulating production of endorphins, producing for most people an increased sense of well-being and neuromuscular relaxation.

Sunshine appears to influence many of the body's hormones. Melatonin, for instance, is produced by the tiny pineal gland deep in the brain and appears to encourage sleep. Sunlight blocks the production of melatonin, which begins to rise only as darkness comes on. The opposite occurs with the hormone cortisone. Natural cortisone is highest in the early morning, and its drop in the evening encourages sleep. These biologic rhythms change only slowly, taking a minimum of five days to reverse. Travelers through three or more time zones can adjust more easily by exposing themselves to light at night and to darkness during the days before travel to hasten their adaptation to a new sleep-wake cycle.

Sunshine stimulus of the thyroid gland increases thyroxine production, which increases body metabolism and burns up more calories, a distinct advantage in weight reduction. Sunlight also acts on the pituitary gland and regulates the sex glands to bring about sexual maturity in children. Children who are blind or otherwise deprived of sunlight tend to reach adolescence earlier than those who have normal eye exposure to sunshine.[18]

Jaundice is a special problem of premature infants. Sunshine (or a sunlamp) alters the bilirubin in the blood of newborns with jaundice so it can be excreted more easily by the kidneys and thus prevent brain damage. A lightly tanned skin gives not only a healthy glow, but also tends to be more resistant to infections and sunburn. However, repeated sunburning is extremely harmful and destroys skin tissue, causing skin to lose its elasticity and protective oil glands. This causes wrinkling and premature aging. Sunburn greatly increases the risk of skin cancer (especially the highly fatal melanomas), which is currently increasing in the U.S. at a rate of 4 percent annually.

Minimal exposure is good, but avoid any exposure which causes burn or deep tanning. This can be done by adequate covering and otherwise avoiding excessive sun exposure or by the use of chemical sunscreens, which absorb the harmful ultraviolet (UV) rays.[19] The UV rays in excessive sunlight are also harmful to eyes— to the cornea, lens, and retina. This is particularly true at high mountain altitudes. Reflected light from snow or water easily burns eyes. UV light and the free radicals it produces are an important stimulant to cataracts. Dark glasses, if they do not absorb UV rays, can do more harm than good. The darkness can cause the pupils to dilate and give even greater exposure to cataract-producing UV rays. UV protection should be built into all eyeglasses, not just sunglasses.

Sunshine is an excellent example of the natural law which says that many things are good in small amounts, but more is not always better. Moderation is an important law of health. Sun provides wonderful benefits, but its favorable effects on health do not require long exposure.

Recreation and Rest

Fatigue is a normal biological reaction to continued physical or mental activity. It is manifested by decreased ability to perform. It can be considered a protective mechanism that prevents the continuation of an activity to the point of irreversible cell damage. Prolonged muscular activity finally leads to a point where muscle will be unable to contract. A thoroughly muscle-fatigued person will be limp and relaxed—hypotonic fatigue. In contrast, a mentally or emotionally fatigued person will exhibit muscle tenseness—hypertonic fatigue. Both will feel equally "tired."

A person's fitness level determines how quickly that person becomes fatigued. A physically unfit person and a tired person both have decreased abilities to perform. More energy is required for any activity and more waste products are produced by that activity; recuperation is prolonged. In a fully rested state, work efficiency is increased, less energy is needed, and less waste produced; fatigue is delayed and recuperation time is shortened.[20]

A major problem occurs in that most people do not distinguish between hypotonic and hypertonic fatigue. The person who has done a hard day of physical labor easily falls asleep with hypotonic fatigue. "The sleep of a laboring man is sweet."[21] The educated person whose work is primarily mental, especially that involving decision making and emotional stress, feels equally tired, but his muscles are tense and sleep does not come easily. His primary need is not sleep but physical exercise to work off the nervous tension. Hypertonic fatigue can become chronic, and chronically fatigued people perform less efficiently. Such people cannot think clearly and soon feel irritable and use poor judgment. As they fall behind in their work, the tendency is to substitute long hours for the inability to perform. "I don't have time to exercise or sleep," they say, without understanding that the only hope of performing better and more efficiently is doing daily physical exercise, thus stimulating healthy sleep.

While the stresses of modern society cannot be avoided entirely, we can help counteract, slow, or lessen their effects. Physical activity that causes the muscles to relax is a tranquilizer that brings rest, sleep, and recuperation. Those who are physically fit and rested can think more clearly and complete more work in less time than those who are not.

The first step to rest is to relax tense muscles. Many people do not know how to relax. Exercise is the best physiological relaxant, but we can otherwise learn to relax through techniques such as these:

> Think of each muscle as a pendulum. The easiest way to get a pendulum to swing to one side is to first pull it to the other side. A muscle will relax more profoundly if you tense it first.

> Lie on your back on a firm surface with your eyes closed. Move around a little until you feel comfortable, then try to lie without moving. Begin by inhaling, tensing your right leg, and raising it a few inches. Hold it for a few seconds, then let it drop as you exhale. Next do the same with your left leg.

> Then inhale deeply and contract the muscles of your right arm as you raise it a few inches off the mat, hold it for about five seconds, and let it drop as you exhale. Do the same with your left arm. Now inhale deeply and contract the muscles of your buttocks as you raise your pelvis off the mat, hold it for about five seconds, and let it drop as you exhale.

> Inhale deeply and push your abdomen out like a balloon, hold your breath for about five seconds, then let your abdomen completely relax as you exhale through your mouth. Repeat the same sequence with your upper chest. Leaving your arms relaxed, inhale and bring your shoulders up toward your ears, then bring them together in front of your chest, and finally push them toward your feet. Relax.

Gently roll your head from side to side and allow your neck to relax. Inhale and squeeze together all of your facial muscles, including your jaw, mouth, eyes, and forehead. Relax. Finally, mentally allow each part of your body to relax even more. While lying there, totally relaxed, observe your breathing. Without trying to change the pattern, just observe or feel the gentle flow of air as it comes in and out of your nose. After a few minutes, allow your inhalations to become a little deeper with each breath. Slowly move your fingers and toes, hands and feet. Then gently roll your arms and legs back and forth. When you are ready, slowly roll over onto your side and come to a seated position.

After you have practiced this deep relaxation several times, you may be able to get into the relaxed state without having to tense and relax each muscle group. For example, simply lie down, inhale deeply, and tense all your muscles simultaneously. Hold this for a few seconds, then release everything as you exhale deeply and relax completely.

After finishing deep relaxation one evening, one participant observed, "It feels like the beginning of the day instead of the end."[22]

Relaxation is a prerequisite to rest and good sleep. Rest, or inactivity, is an important part of life's rhythm and is designed to be regularly interspersed with activity. Regular breaks in your routine enable you to go back to work with renewed vigor. Recreation is vital for all, and *true* recreation restores and helps strengthen a person physically, mentally, and spiritually. Recreation contrasts with amusement, such as inappropriate television viewing, novel reading, and similar activities that occupy and waste time. Remember Paul's admonition not to "share in other people's sins; keep yourself pure."[23]

Sleep, of course, is the best form of rest. It is by no means a passive waste of time. Sleep loss leads to increased irritability, anger, and antisocial behavior; spontaneity disappears, and extended loss of sleep can lead to disorientation, paranoia, depression, and inability to maintain focus on tasks. Perceptiveness and cognitive reasoning abilities decrease. Physically, sleep loss affects the ability to make fine hand movements and focus the eyes; it leads to reduced muscle tone and strength, increased reaction time, and difficulty maintaining good posture. If sleep deprivation continues long enough, death results.

Sleep is divided into two main types: (1) rapid eye movement (**REM**) sleep and (2) non-rapid eye movement (**NREM**) or slow-wave sleep (SWS). Good sleep consists of these two types being interspersed three or four times during the night. Usually SWS predominates during the early hours of sleep and REM during the later hours. Each type serves different important physiological functions.

NREM sleep, which is important for recovery from fatigue, increases after exercise. In this stage, the person is relaxed; blood pressure, respiration, and temperature all decrease; body tone is low; circulation to muscles and organs increases; and blood to the brain decreases. In this stage, the body's physical systems recuperate.

REM sleep is a deep sleep in which the eyes can be observed moving rapidly back and forth. Although asleep, the brain during these times is very active, breathing tends to be irregular, and dreaming occurs. REM sleep appears to restore the nervous system to a resting state and is responsible for establishing mental composure and emotional stability. It is also the time for processing new information in the brain; for instance, transferring material from short-term to long-term memory. REM sleep also affects secretion of several body chemicals, including the cortical steroids. Animals deprived of REM sleep show increased sexual drive, sexual deviance, pleasure and food seeking, and decreased grooming.[24]

People sleep an average of seven or eight hours per night throughout the world, irrespective of the number of hours of daylight present. Several studies seem to confirm that adults who sleep more or less than this tend to have significantly increased death rates. The Alameda County Human Population Study followed a population over nine years. In this study, those who usually slept seven or eight hours each night had significantly lower mortality rates from all disease than respondents reporting six or fewer hours of sleep or those with nine or more hours. Those reporting six or fewer hours of sleep generally experienced the highest death rates. This association between six or fewer (or nine or more) hours of sleep and increased deaths did not appear to be due to differences in physical health status at the beginning of the study.[25]

Although seven or eight hours is a good general recommendation, you should allow your own body to determine how much sleep you need. This is done by going to bed early enough to awaken naturally without an alarm clock.

Alcohol and most sleeping pills disturb normal sleep cycles and especially deprive the body of REM sleep and its restoring effects. Getting sufficient exercise daily and developing a regular sleep schedule are two important aids to good sleep habits. Any exercise done just before going to bed, however, should be light to moderate. Heavy exercise tends to excite the central nervous system and cause sleep disturbances. Studies of college students show that those who have good sleep habits show greater intellectual efficiency, self-control, and sociability. Studies of sailors show that good sleepers fulfill their duties better and tend to be promoted more rapidly.[26]

Other sleep suggestions include having a light, early dinner, or none at all. Digestion increases metabolic activity, making it harder to sleep. Start winding down with relaxing activities at least an hour before bedtime. A warm bath can be helpful. Establish a regular routine.[27] Most important of all, make sure all is right between you and God. Solomon has given this wonderful promise: When you lie down, you will not be afraid; yes, you will lie down and your sleep will be sweet.[28]

Moderation and Self-control

In the parable of the talents (Matthew 25:14-30), Christ taught a principle seen in all nature, a biological law which works in all living things from cell enzymes to large organ systems: Whatever we do not use will be taken from us. In the parable, the man with the single talent did not lose it, nor waste it; he just stored it. Note the climax of the story: "Take the talent from him, and give it to him who has ten talents. For to everyone who has, more will be given, and he will have abundance; but from him who does not have, even what he has will be taken away."[29]

The physical application is clear. Unused muscles atrophy; unstressed bones demineralize; unmoved joints freeze. The less we demand, the less we will have to give. Every function must be judiciously used, or it will be lost—"taken away." Health requires every functional unit of the body to work efficiently—adequately supported and appropriately guided. There are no shortcuts to obtaining and retaining health. No pills, no magic food, no potion from far away. Use the body wisely, or you will lose it in disease and death. It's up to you.

A simple but profound study was initiated by Dr. Lester Breslow while he was director of the California State Health Department. The population of Alameda County was enrolled in a human population study, which began by determining seven health habits or conditions: (1) smoking, (2) drinking alcohol, (3) body weight, (4) exercise, (5) sleep, (6) eating between meals, and (7) breakfast. The habits were categorized as good or bad. Nine years later each health habit was evaluated against the number of deaths that had occurred during that time. The astonishing finding was that in every age category, deaths were directly correlated to the number of good health habits. Those who had more of the good habits had significantly fewer deaths than those who had fewer; the more good habits the better the chance of survival.[30]

It is clear that good health habits relate to health. And just as clear, there are a few things to avoid. Tobacco is the largest preventable cause of adult deaths in the world today. It not only destructs airways and lung tissue, but also promotes cancer in the mouth, larynx, bronchi, and lungs. In the U.S. it causes one-third of heart attacks due to its direct effects on blood vessels and its promotion of atherosclerosis. Not only is it hurtful to the smoker, but it clearly has harmful effects on all those around who are forced to breath the smoke. This particularly includes the children and the spouse of the smoker. Avoid tobacco and do all you can to help others overcome this harmful habit.

All psychoactive chemicals which directly affect the brain should be avoided under normal circumstances. These include alcohol and caffeine-containing drinks. Why carry a handicap when it's not necessary? The brain is too delicate a mechanism to purposely interfere with. Let's support, not destroy our bodies.

God's command for self-control is clear:

> For the grace of God that brings salvation has appeared to all men, teaching us that, denying ungodliness and worldly lusts, we should live soberly, righteously, and godly in the present age, looking for the blessed hope and glorious appearing of our great God and Savior Jesus Christ, who gave Himself for us, that He might redeem us from every lawless deed and purify for Himself His own special people, zealous for good works.[31]

But we don't have to do it in our own strength. Remember this promise:

> Now may the God of peace Himself sanctify you completely; and may your whole spirit, soul, and body by preserved blameless at the coming of our Lord Jesus Christ. He who calls you is faithful, who also will do it.[32]

Healthy Balance

As one considers a healthful lifestyle, it is important to recognize the importance of balance in the body. The chemical constituents of the blood are kept within a very close range (homeostasis). An adequate blood glucose level is vital, and the body works hard to ensure that it does not go too high or too low. Too much of a good thing can be harmful. For example, some exercise is vital, but too much can injure the immune system, making one more prone to infections. It is very important to avoid the tendency to become radical or fanatical about any health practice. The best principle is to maintain a balanced life and develop and grow as did our Example. "And Jesus increased in wisdom and stature, and in favor with God and men."[33] I interpret this to mean that Jesus always balanced mental and physical activity and worshiped God while maintaining good social relations with earthly friends.

Self-control and moderation are important to achieving and maintaining a healthy body. God desires us to have life, not just minimal life, but "abundant life."[34] And God isn't happy with just spiritual health: He encourages a balance.

> Beloved, I pray that you may prosper in all things and be in health, just as your soul prospers.[35]

God is ready to help us worship and glorify Him in our bodies. Living a healthy lifestyle in everything can, by God's grace, lead to greater enjoyment of life. As we give God the credit, we give Him glory. Thanks be to God for His love, grace, and goodness!

[1] Revelation 14:7.

[2] 1 Corinthians 10:31.

[3] Kasch & Boyer, *Adult Fitness: Principles and Practice* (National Press Books, 1968) 16, 17.

[4] Kenneth H. Cooper, *The New Aerobics* (Bantam Books, 1970) 27-34,

[5] Kenneth H. Cooper, *The Aerobics Program for Total Well-Being* (Bantam Books, 1982) 12.

[6] Hebrews 12:1.

[7] 1 Corinthians 9:24.

[8] Dean Ornish, *Eat More, Weigh Less* (Harper, 1993) 46.

[9] Kenneth H. Cooper, *The New Aerobics* (Bantam Books, 1970) 15.

[10] David C. Nieman, D.H.Sc., "Defense in the Best Offense," *Vibrant Life* Sept.-Oct. 1990: 22-25.

[11] W. Raab, MD, *Organized Prevention of Degenerative Heart Disease* (Burlington, VT: Queen City Printers, 1962) 3-7.

[12] Genesis 2:7.

[13] The National Geographic Society, *The Incredible Machine* (1986) 165.

[14] Sebel, Stoddart, et al, *Respiration: the Breath of Life* (Torstar Books, 1985) 95, 96.

[15] The National Geographic Society, Ibid, 166.

[16] David C. Nieman, *The Adventist Healthstyle* (Review & Herald, 1992) 107-109.

[17] Ibid, 109.

[18] Mervyn G. Hardinge, "Sunshine, Friend or Foe?" *Adventist Review* 23 Feb. 1989: 11.

[19] Ludington & Diehl, *Lifestyle Capsules* (Woodbridge Press, 1991) 172, 173.

[20] Mervyn G. Hardinge, *A Philosophy of Health* (School of Health, Loma Linda University, 1980) 15-19.

[21] Ecclesiastes 5:12.

[22] Dean Ornish, MD, *Reversing Heart Disease* (Ballantine Books, 1990) adapted from 162, 163.

[23] 1 Timothy 5:22.

[24] Galen C. Bosley, DHSc, "Sleep," *Ministry* July 1990: 22-24.

[25] Berkman & Breslow, *Health and Ways of Living* (Oxford University Press, 1983) 85, 86.

[26] Galen C. Bosley, Ibid, 24.

[27] Deepak Chopra, "Secrets of Much Better Sleep," *Bottom Line Personal* 1 Feb. 1995: 9, 10.

[28] Proverbs 3:24.

[29] Matthew 25:28, 29.

[30] Berkman & Breslow, *Health and Ways of Living* (Oxford University Press, 1983).

[31] Titus 2:11-14.

[32] I Thessalonians 5:23, 23.

[33] Luke 2:52.

[34] John 10:10.

[35] 3 John 2.

CHAPTER SEVEN

His Judgment Has Come

THE HOUR OF HIS JUDGMENT HAS COME. REVELATION 14:7

The first angel declares, "the hour of His judgment has come."[1] It's a solemn thought that the time has come for the King of the Universe to judge the wicked and justify the righteous. "So then each of us shall give an account of himself to God."[2]

God's standard for judgment is clear. "If you love Me, you will keep my commandments."[3] His commandments include not only the Ten Commandments, but also the physical laws He has created within us. They are closely connected. To intentionally harm our bodies is obviously a violation of the sixth commandment, "Thou shalt not kill."[4] Our love for God causes us to delight in caring for His creation.

Love creates a special relationship with God, one in which we are not afraid of Him as our Judge.

He who has my commandments and keeps them, it is he who loves Me. And he who loves Me will be loved by My Father, and I will love him and manifest Myself to him.[5]

Included within this passage of Scripture is the comforting promise, "Because I live, you will live also."[6] And it's clear that God's desire for us is that we live more than minimal lives. Jesus says, "I have come that they may have life, and that they may have it more abundantly."[7]

The fact that "the hour of His judgment has come" means the time has arrived for everyone to make his final choice for or against God. This is done not so much in large, dramatic decisions as in the small choices we make minute by minute. Do we give glory to God and worship Him in the way we eat, drink, exercise, and rest? Do we wisely use the resources of air, sunshine, and water?

If done from the right motive—to give glory to God, not self—this is holy and righteous living. It is the sanctification that Paul is speaking about when he prays, "Now may the God of peace himself sanctify you completely; and may your whole spirit, soul, and body be preserved blameless at the coming of our Lord Jesus Christ."[8] God is interested in more than our spirit and soul. He sees us as whole beings.

Decision Making

The most awesome gift God gave to the humans created in His image was the ability to think and make choices for themselves. Only a loving God would take the risk of making us capable of rejecting Him. What a measure of His love! True love is never forced; it is always a choice.

The ability to choose, to discriminate between right and wrong, is largely a function of the brain. One author has described the human brain as follows:

> With a brain small enough to be operated on the amount of power that would be needed to burn a 10-watt bulb, man's nervous system in some ways is thousands of times more capable than the most complex calculating machine. Man's comparatively large cerebral cortex gives him better memory, better judgment and better reasoning than any other creature. It permits him to make quicker and more accurate decisions. It provides him with the ability to communicate by speech, to leap intuitively to conclusions that are not clearly indicated by the information he has at hand, and to moderate his body's fight-or-flight reactions by superimposing on primitive emotions such controls as love, joy, understanding, a capability for introspection and a sense of wonder.[9]

Although the brain is increasingly well-mapped, with specific functions known to be located in various portions of the brain, the anatomic location of consciousness, thought, and memory cannot be pinpointed. These higher functions almost certainly involve simultaneous signals in many portions of the cerebral cortex and other areas of the brain, such as the thalamus. The importance of the frontal lobes, however, is evident as we recognize their importance in activities such as controlling choice of behavior in different social or physical situations. The frontal lobes seem to keep the mental functions directed toward goals. They are vital to elaboration of thought, especially the ability to

- predict and plan the future
- delay action in response to incoming sensory signals so that the sensory information can be weighed and the best course of response decided
- consider the consequences of motor actions before they are initiated
- solve complicated mathematical, legal, or philosophical problems
- correlate all avenues of information required to come to a decision, and
- control one's activities in accord with moral laws.[10]

The highest functions of the mind—discrimination, memory, judgment, self-control, and willpower—are the most sensitive to any disturbance in the body. Satan takes advantage of this fact. The path of error usually lies very close to truth, and the devil is a masterful counterfeiter. Satan will in these end times "deceive, if possible, the very elect."[11] He can accomplish this most easily by preventing people from being able to think clearly.

The mind/body interrelationship is too complex to be fully understood. Consciousness and the mind (the brain's thinking portion) are actually functions of the whole body. The brain, the principal organ of the mind and nervous system, is also the master of the body, controlling essentially all functions. At the same time, the brain is totally dependent on such support systems of the body as the digestive, respiratory, circulatory, and excretory systems. When viewed this way, it is clear the human organism is a single unit. We don't just *have* a mind; we *are* a mind—all body tissues support the brain and its function. A castrated male, for example, has a greatly changed personality because of the loss of hormonal balance.[12]

The Devil's Tools to Decrease Ability to Think

The devil very successfully uses many tools to dull the higher brain powers, thus making humans less able to hear the voice of God and discriminate between right and wrong. These include the following:

Lack of oxygen. The central nervous system (CNS) is extremely active, using more oxygen than any other organ. Although the brain is only 3 percent of body weight, it constantly uses 20 percent of the oxygen intake. Anything that interferes with this intake to the CNS dulls the ability of the brain's higher powers. This is brought about by not breathing deeply enough to fully enrich the oxygen-carrying blood, or by disease of the respiratory tract, which interferes with the oxygen/carbon dioxide interchange. It is also illustrated at high altitudes where oxygen pressure is low and where the earliest sign of insufficient oxygen is loss of judgment. Oxygen lack in the brain produces a result similar to the intake of alcohol.

Fatigue. Overwork or loss of sleep manifests itself in increased sluggishness of thought, irritability, and even psychotic-like episodes. A very tired person cannot possibly think clearly.

Nutrition. All have seen the drowsiness that overwhelms a person after eating a heavy meal. The need to bring blood to the gastrointestinal tract to digest the meal deprives the brain of sufficient blood for clear thinking.

Poor diet. Mental disease has been associated with low brain concentration of thiamine (B1), nicotinic acid or nicotinamide (B3), pyridoxine (B6), cyanocobalamin (B12), biotin, ascorbic acid (vitamin C), and folic acid.[13] What you eat does influence how you think!

Poor circulation. Decreased blood supply to the brain prevents clear thinking. Because the rigid skull prevents the brain from expanding, blood vessels in the brain can dilate very little. More than any other organ of the body, the brain is dependent on general circulation. Physical exercise is the best way to increase or improve general circulation and is therefore one of the best ways to clear a mind which has become sluggish due to poor blood supply. Exercise breaks should be mandatory for the desk worker to help keep the mind functioning optimally.

Dehydration. The central nervous system contains more water than any other organ because the multitude of chemical reactions constantly occurring in the brain require water as a medium for their action. Thinking is as much a chemical process as an electrical stimulation. Deprivation of water by drinking too little or losing too much, as in cases of diarrhea or excessive sweating, manifests itself as fatigue, mental apathy, and emotional instability or mental confusion. In addition, chronic or long-term dehydration can lead to kidney failure and severe toxemia (uremia) as body wastes accumulate in the blood.[14]

Toxic conditions. Severe injuries, infections, poisons, and poor function of kidneys or liver all produce mental changes as some of their earliest signs. Restlessness or lethargy, emotional instability, insomnia or drowsiness, and vivid nightmares often appear before other mental changes. Reactions of the body to severe stress are commonly accompanied by loss of ability to think clearly.[15]

Drugs. We are talking here of two main categories: (a) the psychoactive substances commonly taken for their painkilling or tranquilizing effects and (b) the so-called recreational drugs—addicting substances such as tobacco, alcohol, marijuana, and caffeine. Clear thinking is not possible when the body is under the influence of these substances. Judgment, under the influence of drugs, cannot be trusted.

It is significant that even in preparation for the most painful and cruel death imaginable, Jesus refused the vinegar wine offered to Him.[16] I believe Jesus refused the painkiller because He recognized that it would interfere with His ability to think clearly, and thus interfere with His ability to resist the subtle temptations of the devil. His major concern was to maintain clear perception and be able to discriminate between right and wrong as long as He lived.

Attitudes and Emotions and Health

The mind is a physical organ influenced by any change in the body. Anything affecting the circulatory, respiratory, or excretory systems also affects the ability to think. Beyond this, however, even our thoughts influence health and illness. Solomon emphasizes this point:

A merry heart does good, like a medicine, but a broken spirit dries up the bones.[17]

Pleasant words are . . . sweetness to the soul and health to the bones.[18]

This becomes even more meaningful as we remember that it is in the bone marrow that both the immune system white blood cells and the red blood cells are produced. Solomon also reminds us that as a person "thinks in his heart, so is he."[19]

In the New Testament, Paul encourages positive thoughts and emotions.

Rejoice always, pray without ceasing, in everything give thanks; for this is the will of God in Christ Jesus for you.[20]

Finally, brethren, whatever things are true, whatever things are noble, whatever things are just, whatever things are pure, whatever things are lovely, whatever things are of good report, if there is any virtue and if there is anything praiseworthy—meditate on these things.[21]

Norman Cousins has had more influence—even in the scientific world—in helping us understand the relationship between attitudes and health than perhaps any other person. As the former editor of *Saturday Review* and a professor at the University of California School of Medicine, he wrote about his 1964 experience of overcoming a supposedly irreversible collagen disease in a book called *Anatomy of an Illness*. In 1980 he was almost killed by a severe heart attack and wrote of that experience in *The Healing Heart: Antidotes to Panic and Helplessness*. In this second book he tells about his original illness and recovery:

The newspaper accounts had made it appear that I had laughed my way out of a serious illness. Careful readers of my book, however, knew that laughter was just a metaphor for the entire range of the positive emotions. Hope, faith, love, will to live, cheerfulness, humor, creativity, playfulness, confidence, great expectations—all these, I believed, had therapeutic value. Since the negative emotions could set the stage for illness, it seemed to me reasonable to believe that the positive emotions might help set the stage for recovery.

I never regarded the positive emotions, however, as a substitute for scientific treatment. I saw them as providing an auspicious environment for medical care, a method of optimizing prospects of recovery. Another misconception about my illness was that it was a venture in self-care or self-cure. In my book I emphasized the patient-physician partnership.[22]

After describing his recovery from the heart attack, Cousins describes his belief system and philosophy. His major concern is the common feeling of "loss of control" that frequently leads to helplessness and/or panic and its aftermath, depression. He writes,

82

I am inclined to accept the notion that the body produces its own poisons under circumstances of apprehension or emotional strain and that this factor is intimately involved in serious illness, whether it takes the form of cardiac disease, joint disabilities, or even cancer.[23]

He describes how this naturally occurs:

The person who is put on notice by the physician that he or she has a "bad heart" tends to live a life of reduced expectations, to take slower and fewer steps, and to move more tentatively in the outside world. How does one avoid the feeling of being an invalid when underlying conditions create and indeed seem to dictate it?

Perhaps the best way to answer this question is to begin by reflecting on the way the human body works. A weak body becomes weaker in a mood of total surrender. The mechanisms of repair and rehabilitation that are built into the human system have a natural drive to assert themselves (if not discouraged or frustrated). . . . An integral part of this process is respect for the human body—an organism of astounding tenacity, resiliency, and recuperative capability. And, since the human body tends to move in the direction of its expectations—plus or minus—it is important to know that attitudes of confidence and determination are no less a part of the treatment program than is medical science and technology.[24]

The belief that illness is something that comes into us from the outside— a sort of hostile organism or substance that gains entry—is so firmly ingrained in us that we naturally look to available outside forces to do battle with it and evict it. . . . We have little knowledge of, and therefore little confidence in, the numberless ways the human body goes about righting itself. The absence of such knowledge leads . . . to undue fears and even panic, which interferes with the proper functioning of the restorative mechanisms. . . .

Dr. Ingelfinger, the late editor of the New England Journal of Medicine, wrote that about 85 percent of the patients the physician is called upon to treat have self-limiting illnesses. That is, the human body is equipped to meet most of its own health problems. The doctor's job is to distinguish between . . . and to mobilize his knowledge and skills in dealing with the 15 percent. . . .

The notion that the center of the healing process is lodged with the physician is incorrect. It is lodged within the individual, and the wise physician knows how to summon and release it. The individual cannot expect to be relieved of all responsibility in the recovery effort. . . .

What can the individual do? First of all, it is important to be aware of the body's natural drive to heal itself, once freed of the provocations that played a part in bringing on the illness. If a person has a heart attack, for example, the first order of business is to attempt to perceive possible connections between that heart attack and the precipitating causes. If, as in my case, I was engaged in a losing war against congested highways, airport mazes, delayed checkins, overbooked planes, lost luggage, and late lecture arrivals, it was up to me to tame the schedule and make the necessary adjustments. Also, if my body craved exercise it was not receiving, only I was in a position to satisfy that want. And if my physical nourishment had to be augmented with nutrients for the mind, including joyous thoughts and experiences, I could not expect others to meet those needs for me. Each individual presides over the totality of himself or herself—it is imperative that we take on that part of the battle that is uniquely ours. . . .

It is in this sense that we regain control—recognizing the existence of resources represented by the healing system and the belief system that activates it. And the belief system is not just a collection of mechanical parts but a confluence of values and attitudes—hope, faith, confidence, purpose, will to live, and a capacity for joyous living.[25]

Cousins points out that not all illness can be overcome. In cases of serious illness, one should not feel angry or invite defeat. Regeneration works better under some circumstances than others. The factors involved in regeneration include "what we think, what we believe, what we eat, and what we do with our bodies." When disease cannot be reversed, one should not feel that one has failed or that one's "faith and hope were insufficient to our requirements. . . . To feel despair or guilt because we may not always be successful in overcoming illness is to put ourselves above the basic laws of life."[26] He goes on to say that "death becomes tragic only when we have allowed things to die inside us that give meaning to life," and he quotes the physician-philosopher Hans Zinsser, who describes what he learned in his final illness:

My mind is more alive and vivid than ever before. My sensitivities are keener; my affections stronger. I seem for the first time to see the world in clear perspective. I love people more deeply and comprehensively. I seem to be just beginning to learn my business and see my work in its proper relationship to science as a whole. I seem to myself to have entered into a period of stronger feelings and saner understanding.[27]

With the right attitude, there is much to learn and experience even while approaching death. Cousins summarizes the things he experienced that he feels might help others, recognizing that what worked for him might not work for everyone. Here are his main points:

- First, conquest of panic is an essential part of recovery from a serious disease. Confidence, deep purpose, joyousness, laughter, and the will to live are good conditioning agents in this conquest and recovery.

- Second, while the body's drive to recuperate may not always work, it works often enough to warrant one's confidence and special effort.

- Third, sharing responsibility with one's physician is in the best interests of both physician and patient.

- Fourth, there may be times when surgery can be avoided, but there is never a time when the nourishment one puts into one's body or one's mind is not essential to health.

- Fifth, when faced with surgical or other heavy interventions, don't hesitate to get a second or third opinion. Whether the body can recover without such interventions requires the greatest wisdom available.

- Sixth, medical treatment should seek not just to repair damage and restore vital balances but to enhance the quality of life and help the patient overcome feelings of hopelessness and helplessness. The patient must be a responsible and appreciative partner.

A happy and optimistic outlook on life has been shown to contribute directly to a healthier immune system. Recent studies show this is brought about neurologically and is not entirely psychologic.[28]

The Ultimate Function of the Brain

The knowledge that we live in the time of judgment forces us to face the consequences of our choices. Satan dulls our minds in many ways and prevents people from discriminating clearly between right and wrong. We must give the highest priority to helping our bodies maintain clear minds.

The devil also works to influence our attitudes. He attempts to overwhelm us with guilt, worry, anger, depression, and other negative thoughts. With God's help we must counteract this with positive attitudes and emotions, such as love, joy, peace, and confidence and faith in God. Such thinking is necessary for health, healing, and stronger immune systems.

The brain's highest function, however, is to be the dwelling place, through His Spirit, of Jesus Himself. Within the highest center of the brain is a mysterious place in which Christ desires to dwell. Although it cannot be pinpointed anatomically, it is a physical place where Jesus stands outside and knocks, waiting for us to invite Him in.[29] When accepted and invited in, He is "Christ in you, the hope of glory."[30]

Prayer

Dear Lord, only with Your help can I resist the constant effort of Satan to overcome me. Only You can give both physical and spiritual victory and enable me to face unafraid my Father, the final Judge of all things. The angel's message, that the "hour of His judgment has come," is a call to recommit my life to You. With Your help, every choice I make in the struggle of life can be directed and blessed by You. Thank you, Lord, for the reminder of my need and opportunity to live a happy and holy life! Amen.

---

[1] Revelation 14:7.

[2] Romans 14:12.

[3] John 14:15 (marginal reference).

[4] Exodus 20:13 (KJV).

[5] John 14:21.

[6] John 14:19.

[7] John 10:10.

[8] I Thessalonians 5:23.

[9] Alan E. Nourse, LIFE Science Library: *The Body* (Time-Life Books, 1964) 150.

[10] Arthur C. Guyton, MD, *Human Physiology and Mechanisms of Disease* (W.B. Saunders, 1987) 419.

[11] Matthew 24:24.

[12] Stanley Cobb in "Mind-Body Relationships," Lief, Lief & Lief, eds., *The Psychological Basis of Medical Practice* (Harper and Row, Hoeber Medical Division, 1963) 36-43.

[13] Charles Gerras, ed., *The Complete Book of Vitamins* (Rodale Press, 1977) 337.

[14] Briggs & Calloway, *Nutrition and Physical Fitness, 11th ed.* (Holt, Rinehart & Winston, 1984) 318, 319.

[15] Beeson, McDermott, & Wyngaarden, *Cecil's Textbook of Medicine,* Asian ed. (W.B. Saunders, 1979), 647.

[16] Matthew 27:34; Mark 15:23.

[17] Proverbs 17:22.

[18] Proverbs 16:24.

[19] Proverbs 23:7.

[20] 1 Thessalonians 5:16-18.

[21] Philippians 4:8.

[22] Norman Cousins, *The Healing Heart: Antidotes to Panic and Helplessness* (W. W. Norton & Co, 1983) 50, 51.

[23] Cousins, Ibid, 242.

[24] Ibid, 222, 223.

[25] Ibid, 227- 230.

[26] Ibid, 230, 231.

[27] Hans Zinsser, *As I Remember Him* (Little Brown, 1940).

[28] David S. McKinsey, MD, *Healing Unlimited* (Boardroom Classics, 1995) 2.

[29] Revelation 3:20.

[30] Colossians 1:27.

CHAPTER EIGHT

Babylon is Fallen

AND ANOTHER ANGEL FOLLOWED, SAYING, "BABYLON IS FALLEN, IS FALLEN, THAT GREAT CITY, BECAUSE SHE MADE ALL NATIONS DRINK OF THE WINE OF THE WRATH OF HER FORNICATION." REVELATION 14:8.

The second angel proclaims the good news, "Babylon is fallen, is fallen."[1] How comforting it should be to know the enemy is defeated and sin has been conquered! When Christ on the cross cried, "It is finished,"[2] He was announcing that Satan was vanquished. Unfortunately, most people choose to stay in Babylon, and many don't know they serve a defeated enemy. God is forced to give a special message, "Come out of her (Babylon), my people, lest you share in her sins, and lest you receive of her plagues."[3]

Confusion (Babylon) began in the Garden of Eden when Eve and Adam chose to follow their personal inclinations rather than God's will. The overwhelming temptation was that they might become "like God, knowing good and evil," and when Eve saw that the fruit was "desirable to make one wise," she took, ate, gave to her husband, and he ate.[4] The evil effects of human desires and distrust of God began here.

Currently there are almost six billion self-centered humans on earth, each seeking to be his or her own "god." Promoting personal desire is one of Satan's most successful ploys. In a world where selfishness rules, confusion naturally follows. How wonderful to know that we don't have to stay in Babylon. God is longing for us to choose His peace, not Satan's confusion. God offers,

Peace I leave with you, My peace I give to you; not as the world gives do I give to you. Let not your heart be troubled, neither let it be afraid.[5]

Self-esteem Movement

Satan's confusion is seen in modern thinking, which includes the belief that if it feels good or tastes good, it must *be* good; therefore, live by your feelings. Babylon's confusion also challenges us to develop the power within, to improve our own selves. The modern self-esteem movement in the United States illustrates this thinking. As with all counterfeits, "self-esteem" has so much truth and value that it is difficult not to be misled by false teaching.

The command to "Love your neighbor as yourself" is a reminder we must value self in order to love others.[6] We need to remember, however, that self-worth is not really self-created. Individual value is measured by the unconditional love of God that led Jesus to die for sinners. "God demonstrates His own love toward us, in that while we were still sinners, Christ died for us."[7] "Whoever does not practice righteousness is not of God, nor is he who does not love his brother. . . . Because He laid down His life for us, we also ought to lay down our lives for the brethren."[8] Jesus lived a perfect example of unselfishness.

Newsweek ran a cover story entitled "The Curse of Self-Esteem: What's Wrong With the Feel-Good Movement." It contained a thought-provoking report of the confusion of modern Babylon in the fields of religion, education, and business. My summary of this article follows:

> As a concept, self-esteem can be traced to Freud, who used the term ego *ideal*, but it has now become a way of trying to make sense of the wildly proliferating addictions and dependencies of our time. People were hoping they could find one solution to many problems.

> **Churches** have discovered that "low self-esteem" is less offensive to congregations than "sin." Americans seem partial to such naive optimism as "Every day in every way I am getting better and better."

> Many churches now teach that sin is more "not living up to one's own potential" than the breaking of God's commandments. There's no sense that you broke some law or rule and that you're not good enough. Chastising sinners is considered counterproductive because it makes them feel worse about themselves.

> Nowhere has the self-esteem concept taken root as firmly as in **education**. Toddlers are encouraged to "reach their full potential" in daycare centers. Some schools abolish failing grades to avoid hurting children. Trophies are given just for attending a sports event.

> Of course children need encouragement, but "praise has to be connected with values, with the development of character. Kids need authentic feed-back, not praise for walking across the room without falling over." But most teachers do not want to wait for children to do something right when it's so much simpler just to praise them all the time.

> Self-esteem does not necessarily translate into better scholastic perfor-mance. Harold Stevenson, a psychologist at the University of Michigan, recently found that American schoolchildren rank far ahead of students in Japan, Taiwan, and China in self-confidence about their abilities in math.

Unfortunately, this is marred by the fact that Americans are far behind in *actual performance* in math. In math and science achievement, compared with 20 other countries, American schoolchildren rank near the bottom. It appears that Americans put too much emphasis on "being happy."

An Atlanta school principal, Jacqueline Ponder, says, "Once they have their self-esteem, they don't need anything else. They *are*. And all they have to do is develop that which they are." It is less a matter of scientific pedagogy than of faith—faith that positive thoughts can make manifest the inherent goodness in anyone, even 10-year-old boys.

Businesses have begun to realize that improving employees' self -esteem, usually known in this context as "empowerment," can be a more effective motivator than expensive, old fashioned "raises." "Self-esteem is a basic building block on which personal effectiveness is based," says Dave Ehlen, a management-training consultant with Wilson Learning Corporation. Even America's corporate managers, whose excessive salaries have become something of a national scandal, must be made to "believe in themselves . . . to feel good about what they are and where they are going."

From cradle to grave, Americans are being urged to feel good about themselves and to reach for their full potential. This is despite the lack of scientific evidence of any direct relationships between lack of self-esteem and drug abuse, substance abuse, crime and violence, or teen pregnancy. In fact, relating to the latter, two studies linked *high* self-esteem with increased sexual activity by teens.[9]

The "feel-good" movement is mostly an American phenomenon, and a British viewpoint is given in an accompanying article. Carol Sarler suggests that the "national obsession with this thing called 'self-esteem' is a reaction of the U.S. to the end of the Cold War and the necessity to do something to make everyone feel better at no risk. She makes some good points in saying it is actually evidence of immaturity. To Americans she says,

None of these differences, by themselves, can explain the distaste and alarm with which we view your current mission to feel better about yourselves. This mission is actually dangerous. Your quest is the stuff of childhood. It is part of the growing process to explore the self and soul, to discover how to relate to others, to learn to love and to be loved, to gain in confidence . . . while a firmer hand rocks your cradle. And it is the stuff of childhood precisely because it is not compatible with adult responsibility. . . .

When you are the most powerful nation in the world, it is too late to have a childhood of any description. And regardless of the recent blows to the collective American ego, you are still a people whose votes affect the world and whose leaders run it—which is why the rest of us need you to get it right in the most adult and the most responsible way possible. Without feeling good, if necessary.

Frankly, we do not wish you to become infused with self-esteem; we would feel more comfortable—not to mention a mite safer—if you opted for self doubt. . . . You know what I'm saying? Just grow up.[10]

Immaturity, the belief that the purpose of life is to feel good, has many negative side effects. It is the result of selfish thinking—placing self above God or others.

Selfishness

While selfishness is at the root of the sins of Babylon, it has been publicly emphasized only recently. At the turn of the twentieth century, there was little idea of putting oneself first. Emphasis was much stronger on community values; one's first duty was to family, friends, and community. James Lincoln Collier describes the recent increase in selfishness:

After World War I, people began feeling they wanted to have a free, expressive life. Gradually, this became translated into a sense that they should feel good all the time. By the 1970s this became an actual ethic that said you were wrong if you weren't putting yourself first. . . . In the early 1970s, self indulgence just went through the roof. The figures jumped tremendously for drinking, for teenage sex, for premarital pregnancy, for drug use. The economic boom that followed World War II caused children to grow to adulthood assuming they should have whatever they wanted.

Television has had its influence. The current generation grew up seeing, on an average, 20,000 irresponsible commercial messages each year—each designed to make one feel a desire for material things. Without a doubt, Americans are spending lots of money on things they really don't need. Two billion dollars a year is spent on pornographic phone calls and we pay some baseball players as much as $5 million a year. At a time we are spending $170 billion a year for primary and secondary education for our children, we are spending $150 billion a year for illegal drugs. A few years ago, the Bush administration got excited about the war on drugs and scrambled desperately to find $10 billion to fight drugs. That same year, Americans spent $21 billion for pizza. Does it make sense?

The abandonment of children is the most serious symptom of selfishness. We feel we have a right to have children and then we put them in day-care centers. We don't even try to give them two parent homes. Twenty-five percent of all children born in the U.S. (40 percent in New York City) are born into fatherless homes. But no one's willing to say to couples, *Look, you've got to stay married. If you've got kids, stay married.* That marriage is sometimes boring is not the point; the point is that sometimes we have to do things for the good of our children and those around us instead of looking for our own gratification.

Not taking full responsibility for our children affects their behavior and view of life. Putting young children in day-care centers may not be good for them. They tend to quickly become very good socially with their peers and less interested in what their parents think or ask them to do. They tend not to take orders from adults well.[11]

Breakup of the Family

I believe in the symbolic interpretation of Revelation 14, but I consider it no accident that the Revelator calls the sin of Babylon *fornication*, also translated as *adulteries, impure passion, intense impurity,* and *passionate immorality.* Lustful appetite is a special temptation in this end time; it leads to violence at home and the breakup of the family. Children particularly suffer.

In 1994 more than one million cases of child abuse and neglect were confirmed in the U.S., an increase of 27 percent since 1990. The report "Child Maltreatment 1994" found that 53 percent of maltreated children suffered neglect, 26 percent physical abuse, 14 percent sexual abuse, 5 percent emotional abuse, and 22 percent other forms of maltreatment. Nearly half of the abused children were six years old or younger. Estimates of the problem's actual extent are hard to obtain. Preliminary results of the "Third National Incidence Study of Child Abuse and Neglect" indicate that actual maltreatment victims may number almost three times higher than shown in state reports.[12]

An estimated 462,000 children were found to be in substitute or foster care, nearly twice as many as a decade ago, and 1,300 children died as a result of their abuse. But the problem doesn't end there. Children who live in abusive families to the age of eight or ten risk becoming so emotionally and psychologically damaged that they can never be repaired; they tend to perpetuate their trauma into the next generation.[13] The problem is so bad that *U.S. News & World Report* devoted two cover stories to it in less than 12 months.[14] Evidence shows that it is a world-wide problem, not just an American one.

U.S. divorce rates doubled between 1965 and 1976 and have continued to increase since. In 1990, 1,175,000 couples were divorced, with 1,045,750 children involved. Studies indicate children of divorce have a higher chance of getting divorced themselves. A 1987 study at the University of Texas found that white women younger than 16 when their parents divorced or separated were 59 percent more likely to get divorced or separated themselves. A study of 60 divorced couples in California found that almost half of their children "entered adulthood as worried, underachieving, self-deprecating and sometimes angry young men and women."[15]

Breakup of marriage is a problem among Christians even as among non-Christians. What can be done? John Gottman, professor of psychology at the University of Washington, suggests after studying more than 2,000 couples for more than two decades that he can predict a marriage's prospects with 94 percent accuracy. His study indicates the following significant warning signs:

- If your marriage doesn't have a ratio of five positive interactions or periods of time for every negative one, it is less likely to last. For instance, if a couple has a nasty falling out that lasts for a half hour, a winning couple needs to spend two and one-half hours reconciling and making up.
- It is a danger when one slips from complaining (a more okay trait) to criticizing. For instance, the accusation is made, "You just never call when you're going to be late," instead of the more neutral "I wish you'd call me when you're going to be late."
- If a couple can't clearly recollect details of their courtship, their marriage is in jeopardy.
- Nothing foretells a marriage's future as accurately as how a couple retell the experiences of their marriage. Couples who stay together tend to have the attitude, "We can survive anything."
- Husbands' responses are more predictive than those of the wives. Men tend to display signs of marital distress earlier and more intensely than women.
- A sign of irreversible failure in marriage is a process called "flooding." When a man's heart goes up to 80 beats per minute (normal 72-76), or a woman's rises to 90 beats per minute, flooding begins. At this level the physiological arousal makes it hard for one partner to focus on what the other person is saying and leads to defensiveness and hostility.[16]

Gottman suggests that the number one thing to do if you have any negative symptoms is to "work out a comfortable, effective way of dealing with your differences. . . ." By being more open, "you can learn to inoculate your relationship against the stresses that can lead to divorce. After a while, the behavior becomes automatic."[17]

A timely issue of the *Adventist Review* published in 1993 was entitled "Sexual Misconduct: Abusing a Precious Gift." It points out that Seventh-day Adventists are not immune from the sins of the family. "It's time," the editor writes, "for all sexual abuse of children to stop. Jesus pronounced the sternest warning against anyone who violates the innocence of a child.[18] It's time for everyone in a position of authority to examine his or her ways lest we cross over into the forbidden zone in sexual relationships. It's time to put away the sins of the family."[19]

In that same issue, Karen Flowers writes of "Human Sexuality: God's Bright Thread of Joy." Bible writers, she points out, unabashedly worshiped God with mind, spirit, and body.[20] When God completed the creation of man and woman, He pronounced it not good, but "very good."[21] Jesus affirmed God's positive view of sexuality.[22] Human sexuality is the metaphor used to describe the desired intimacy between God and human beings. The imagery of marriage, which in Scripture always implies sexual union, enriches the New Testament understanding of Christ as the bridegroom and the church as the cherished bride.[23]

"Wives, submit to your own husbands, as to the Lord. For the husband is head of the wife"[24] is often cited by abusive husbands to justify their behavior. The word *submit*, however, does not occur in the original Greek. *Mutual* submission is the point. A husband is to love his wife as his own body. "Be subject to one another out of reverence for Christ"[25] is the principle behind this passage.[26]

Marriage counselors are vulnerable to sexual exploitation of their clients. Peter Rutter estimates that 10 percent of male psychotherapists have had sexual contact with at least one client. Len McMillan, director of church ministries for the Potomac Conference of Seventh-day Adventists, reports that 12.5 percent of 586 respondents, mostly Adventist pastors, indicated in a survey that they had had an affair.[27] How can professional abuse be prevented?

- First, ongoing educational programs that teach sexual ethics must be presented to caregivers.

- Second, people needing professional counsel should be aware of warning signs of possible misconduct—excessive self-disclosure of the counselor's marital problems, sex brought up out of context, or the client just having a gut feeling that something is *really not right.28*

Finally, it is important to remember the Bible's injunction:

Brothers, if someone is caught in a sin, you who are spiritual should restore him gently. But watch yourself, or you also may be tempted. Carry each other's burdens, and in this way you will fulfill the law of Christ.[29]

Women's Health

Women especially suffer from the selfishness of Babylon. Largely due to neglect, more than half a million women (at least 90 percent of them from the developing world) die each year in pregnancy or childbirth—an average of one a minute. The astonishing contrast between the rich and poor nations is that 600 mothers per 100,000 live births die in Africa; 400 in Asia; 300 in Latin America; and 10 in Northern Europe and North America.[30] In other words, the chance of maternal mortality in Africa is one in 20; in the U.S. it is one in 6,366.[31]

This intolerably large gap between women in the developing world and women in industrialized societies is due to many things: lack of adequate medical care, neglect of female children, early marriages, poverty, lack of female education and high illiteracy, overwork, and underfeeding. Affluent women in North America and Europe devote approximately 14 percent of their life spans to reproduction, in contrast to many women in the developing world who devote 50 percent of their shorter life spans to this task. Women who are frequently pregnant are in a constant state of fatigue. For every woman who dies there are 15 chronically disabled. Half the mothers who die, according to some studies, had unwanted pregnancies.[32]

A survey of women's groups from developing countries in the late 1980s found violence the top common concern. Anthropologists confirm that if there is anything universal about the female condition, it is vulnerability to assault.[33] Women in the U.S. have a one in four risk of being raped, and girls have a greater than one in three risk of sexual abuse by an adult. Other studies reveal that 40 to 50 percent of women have experienced some form of sexual harassment.[34]

The July 4, 1994, cover story of *Newsweek* was entitled "Battered Women: Living in Terror." It reports that 1,400 women are killed in the U.S. by their spouses each year, while about two million are beaten—on average, one every 16 seconds. The Surgeon General of the U.S. reports that for women between 15 and 44, domestic abuse is the leading cause of injury.

A *U. S. News & World Report* cover story states that "in much of the world, political and economic 'progress' has been dragging women backward," and suggests that "women are falling further behind in country after country—and their men like it that way."[35]

The horrible result of the devil having his way in this world is clear. Our gracious God pleads, "Come out of her, my people, lest you share in her sins, and receive of her plagues."[36]

AIDS is a modern plague claiming many women and children. About 10 percent of those with AIDS are infants and children under the age of five. The pandemic is worldwide, but especially hard hit are the ten countries of Central and East Africa, where it is estimated that up to three million women will die of this devastating disease during the 1990s. In these same countries, by the year 2000, we can expect 5.5 million children under the age of 15 to be orphaned by the disease. Grandmothers who would normally count upon sons to provide for their old age are instead burying their adult offspring and caring for seven to ten or more parentless children. Most grandmothers have no means and little strength to do so.[37]

Wine of Babylon

While we cannot ignore the symbolism in Revelation 14, a look at its literal language provides us a vivid description of modern problems. One of the devil's most successful ploys is to get humans to deaden their thinking ability with alcoholic drinks. Easily made from any starchy substance, alcohol is almost universally available through home brews or commercial breweries or distilleries. As mentioned in a previous chapter, alcohol is pharmaceutically an anesthetic; it begins by dulling the highest powers of the mind—judgment, discrimination, and will-power.

Use of alcohol is increasing in the developing world. The World Health Organization reports that if present trends continue, per capita consumption of alcohol in many developing countries will equal or surpass that of the West in less than a generation. Already, alcohol-induced cirrhosis of the liver is one of Mexico's leading causes of death among men ages 25 to 54. Eleven percent of adult Mexican males are addicted to alcohol. In Chile, reports show alcohol directly or indirectly involved in 53 percent of all deaths. In Trinidad and Tobago, 47 percent of males admitted to the country's largest hospital have medical problems related to drinking. Post-mortem studies reveal that one-third to one-half of accident victims in developing countries are legally drunk at the time of the crash.

Increasingly the demand for alcohol causes food to be diverted to alcohol production, often causing food shortages. As much as one-third of malnutrition in some areas can be attributed to the father's drinking habit, although alcohol is seldom mentioned as a factor in child health.[38]

More than half of all adults detained in U.S. jails and prisons have addictive disorders. Juveniles detained by the justice system are more than twice as likely as their peers to use alcohol and other drugs heavily, and two-thirds have parents with addictive disorders. Nearly one in three high school seniors "binge drink" (consume five or more drinks in a row); 13 percent of eighth graders report binge drinking.

About 9 percent of adult Americans—15.2 million people—are alcoholics. It is much higher in many other countries. One in 10 American women at peak reproductive age (18 to 34) drinks enough alcohol (two or more drinks per day) to expose an unborn child to the potential of birth defects. Substance abuse is tied to violence and accidental injury on the job, on the highway, and in the home. It plays a significant role in child abuse, rape, lost productivity, and increased medical costs to society.[39]

Summary

The statistics reveal the evil results of Babylon's sins. Despite the harmful effects, many are still attracted to alcohol and lust of the flesh. I believe God, by using such descriptive language in the second angel's message, is seeking to make people aware of the special temptations of this age. Thank God His people don't stay under the spell of fallen Babylon. God is calling all to come out, and He pleads, "Do not be conformed to this world, but be transformed by the renewing of your mind, that you may prove what is that good and acceptable and perfect will of God."[40]

What a contrast God's plan is to the wine of the wrath of her fornication that Babylon forces all to drink. The symbolism of the second angel's message has serious implications when interpreted literally. Selfish living is destructive of body, mind, and soul. God, help us to understand this and come out of Babylon.

---

[1] Revelation 14:8.

[2] John 19:30.

[3] Revelation 18:4.

[4] Genesis 3:5, 6.

[5] John 14:27.

[6] Leviticus 19:18; Romans 13:9.

[7] Romans 5:8.

[8] 1 John 3:10, 16.

[9] Jerry Adler, et al, "Hey, I'm Terrific," *Newsweek* 17 Feb. 1992: 46-51.

[10] Carol Sarler, "Stiffen Your Lips, Yanks; No Self-esteem, Please, We're British," *Newsweek* 17 Feb. 1992: 52.

[11] James Lincoln Collier, "The Rise of Selfishness," *Bottom Line Personal* 30 April 1992: 11, 12.

[12] "New HHS Report Shows Increase in Child Abuse," APHA: *The Nation's Health* May/June 1996: 4, 8.

[13] Ingrassia & McCormick, "Why Leave Children With Bad Parents?" *Newsweek* 25 April 1994: 52-58.

[14] "Unlocking Hidden Memories: Can 'Forgotten' Childhood Abuse Come Back to Haunt You Years Later?" *U. S. News & World Report* 29 Nov. 1993: 52-64 and "Sexual Predators: Can They Be Stopped?" *U. S. News & World Report* 19 Sept. 1994: 64-76.

[15] Barbara Kantrowitz, et al, "The Legacy of Divorce: Breaking the Divorce Cycle," *Newsweek* 13 Jan. 1992: 48-53.

[16] Linda Murray, "Can Divorce Be Predicted?" *Longevity* Aug. 1994: 32 and 70-72.

[17] Ibid, 72.

[18] Matthew 18:6-10.

[19] William G. Johnsson, "Sins of the Family," *Adventist Review* 2 Sept. 1993: 4.

[20] Psalm 63:1; 84:1, 2; Romans 8:23; 1 Corinthians 6:12-20.

[21] Genesis 1:31.

[22] Matthew 19:3-12.

[23] Karen Flowers, "Human Sexuality: God's Bright Thread of Joy," *Adventist Review* 2 Sept. 1993.

[24] Ephesians 5:22.

[25] Ephesians 5:22 (RSV).

[26] Ron Flowers, "A Christian Response to Intimate Violence," *Adventist Review* 2 Sept. 1993.

[27] H. Susi Mundy, "Behind Closed Doors: Mutual Consent or Abuse of Power?" *Adventist Review* 2 Sept. 1993.

[28] Ibid, 15.

[29] Galatians 6:1, 2 (NIV).

[30] Lettenmaier, Liskin, Church, and Harris, "Mothers' Lives Matter: Maternal Health in the Community," *Population Reports,* Population Information Program, Johns Hopkins University, Sept. 1988: 2.

[31] Naomi Baumslag, MD, "Barriers to Women's Health, Nutrition and Status: A Global Perspective," *Interface,* ADRA International, vol 8, no. 2, 1991: 5.

[32] Ibid.

[33] Emily MacFarqhar, "The War Against Women," *U. S. News & World Report* 28 Mar. 1994: 45.

[34] David R. Williams, "Why Does Sexual Abuse Occur?" *Adventist Review* 2 Sept. 1993: 18.

[35] *U. S. News & World Report* 28 March 1994.

[36] Revelation 18:4.

[37] *Children and AIDS: An Impending Calamity* (New York: UNICEF, 1990).

[38] Lori Heise, "Trouble Brewing: Alcohol in the Third World," *World Watch* July-Aug. 1991: 11-18.

[39] "Making Prevention & Treatment Work," Substance Abuse and Mental Health Services Administration, DHHS Publication No. (SMA) 93-2058, 1993.

[40] Romans 12:2.

CHAPTER NINE

If Anyone Worships the Beast

THEN A THIRD ANGEL FOLLOWED, SAYING WITH A LOUD VOICE, "IF ANYONE WORSHIPS THE BEAST AND HIS IMAGE, AND RECEIVES HIS MARK ON HIS FOREHEAD OR ON HIS HAND, HE HIMSELF SHALL ALSO DRINK OF THE WINE OF THE WRATH OF GOD, WHICH IS POURED OUT FULL STRENGTH INTO THE CUP OF HIS INDIGNATION. HE SHALL BE TORMENTED WITH FIRE AND BRIMSTONE IN THE PRESENCE OF THE HOLY ANGELS AND IN THE PRESENCE OF THE LAMB. AND THE SMOKE OF THEIR TORMENT ASCENDS FOREVER AND EVER." REVELATION 14:9-11

What a graphic description of the final results of false worship and sin! This should be understood as an outworking of the principle Paul taught the Galatians:

Do not be deceived, God is not mocked; for whatever a man sows, that he will also reap. For he who sows to the flesh will of the flesh reap corruption. . . .[1]

The Final Results of Sin

God's judgments are mostly the natural results of our poor choices: "For the wages of sin is death."[2] The devil tries to convince us otherwise. In Eden God said, "of every tree of the garden you may freely eat; but of the tree of the knowledge of good and evil you shall not eat, for in the day that you eat of it *you shall surely die*."[3] But through the serpent the devil said, "You will *not* surely die."[4] This has been through the centuries one of Satan's most convincing lies. The belief in the immortality of the soul, its transmigration into other beings, and communication with spirits (spiritualism) are all the logical follow-up of the lie perpetrated in Eden, "You will not surely die."

The best interpretation of "in the day that you eat of it you shall surely die" is that on the day you die spiritually, you begin to die physically. The cells of mortal man are constantly dying. Fortunately there is also the process of regeneration, except in the nervous system. Nerve cells that die—or those that are killed by toxins such as anesthetics or alcohol—do not regenerate. Aging is slow death, but the good news is that good health habits and the blessing of God can postpone or delay our death sentence.

Jesus speaks of death as sleep.[5] In fact, the Bible speaks of death as sleep more than 50 times. The wise man, Solomon, reminds us that "the living know that they will die; but the dead know nothing."[6] Only God has immortality.[7] Although the Bible speaks of *soul* at least 1,600 times, not once does it speak of *immortal soul*. Man became a "living soul" when God breathed into him the "breath of life."[8] We await the second coming of Jesus when He will give us immortality.[9]

A common misunderstanding involves the eternal punishment of the wicked. Revelation says, "the smoke of their torment ascends forever and ever."[10] Malachi makes clear that in that last day the wicked will be as "stubble" and will "burn up," while the righteous "shall trample the wicked, for they shall be as ashes under the soles of your feet."[11] The Psalmist points out that the wicked shall "be no more." They will "vanish away" and will not be found.[12] The earth and the results of sin will be "dissolved" and "melt with fervent heat," but "the new earth" and the New Jerusalem will come down to the cleansed earth.[13] It does not come down into a continually burning fire, for the righteous do not walk around in fire.

Sodom and Gomorrah suffered "the vengeance of *eternal fire*,"[14] but they are not still burning. Jesus speaks of hell as having fire "that shall never be quenched,"[15] just as the destruction of Jerusalem was predicted as occurring with fire that "shall not be quenched."[16] History tell us that Jerusalem was destroyed by Titus in AD 70 by a fire that could not be put out, but it is not burning now. Eternal fire refers to fire that cannot be put out until it has accomplished its purpose, God's judgment on sin and sinners. "They shall be as though they had never been."[17] Isaiah explains that the wicked shall burn as stubble; they cannot "deliver them-selves from the power of the flame"; but eventually there shall not "be a coal to be warmed by, nor a fire to sit before."[18] Sin will be no more and the earth will be eternally cleansed from any trace of sin. Praise God!

Although God's judgment results from our poor choices, God in His mercy has often softened the consequences. "The Lord is . . . longsuffering toward us, not willing that any should perish."[19] This was illustrated many times toward the children of Israel as they traveled toward Canaan. At the time of Jonah's mission, it was said of Ninevah that "God relented from the disaster that He had said He would bring upon them, and He did not do it."[20] God is "rich in mercy, because of His great love with which He loved us,"[21] and this longsuffering was seen in the way He waited patiently for the antideluvians in the days of Noah.[22]

It is really God's love and mercy that forces sin to its final conclusion. It is merciful to let death come to those who have chosen an unhappy life by their refusal to worship and trust God. God lets us experience the results of sin ourselves; moreover, by faith we can come to know Christ and His suffering for us as the result of our sin. When we recognize the horror of sin so strongly that we will never be tempted to sin again, the great controversy will be over. Heaven is immune to sin because of the vaccination to the disease of sin we receive here on earth.

True Worship

False worship of the "beast and his image"[23] and the results of receiving his "mark" are painted graphically to encourage us to reject false worship. In this treatise we choose not to go into the theology of the beast and his image, other than to recognize the concept of false worship. The positive approach to the third angel's message is to seek an understanding of true worship.

Worship is "respect, reverence paid to a divine being."[24] True worship of God can be placed under three headings: (1) **communion with God**, (2) **use of our bodies in worship**, and (3) **worship in action** (practical worship).

Communion with God. We show our love and respect to God by our constant communion with Him. Paul encourages us to "pray without ceasing."[25] "Be anxious for nothing, but in everything by prayer and supplication, with thanksgiving, let your requests be made known to God; and the peace of God which surpasses all understanding, will guard your hearts and minds through Christ Jesus."[26] David suggests that prayer is by word and meditation: "Let the words of my mouth and the meditation of my heart be acceptable in Your sight, O Lord, my strength and my Redeemer."[27]

Paul speaks to Timothy about being "sanctified by the word of God and prayer."[28] The word of God should be the ultimate subject of our prayers. "Your word I have hidden in my heart, that I might not sin against you. . . . Your word is a lamp to my feet and a light to my path."[29] "For the word of God is living and powerful, and sharper than any two-edged sword, piercing even to the division of soul and spirit, and of joints and marrow, and is a discerner of the thoughts and intents of the heart."[30] Through God's Word and by inspiration of the Holy Spirit, humans can overcome in common temptations and develop a worshipful relationship with God. This is maintained only by continuous prayer and meditation.

Use of our bodies in worship. "Do you not know that your body is the temple of the Holy Spirit, who is in you, whom you have from God, and you are not your own? For you were bought at a price; therefore glorify God in your body and in your spirit, which are God's."[31] This was emphasized in Chapter 3, where the first angel's message commanded that we "give glory . . . and worship Him who made heaven and earth, the sea and springs of water."[32] Paul pleads, "I beseech [urge] you therefore, brethren, by the mercies of God, that you present your bodies a living sacrifice, holy, acceptable to God, which is your reasonable service [spiritual worship, RSV]."[33]

One way to serve God is to live holy lives in the bodies He has given us. That means we must give up (sacrifice) our natural, unholy tendencies and desires; however, this is not by our own effort. "I can do all things through Christ who strengthens me."[34] Only in this way can we "be transformed by the renewing of your mind [so we] may prove what is that good and acceptable and perfect will of God."[35]

Worship in action. "Is not this the fast [worship] that I have chosen: to loose the bonds of wickedness, to undo the heavy burdens, to let the oppressed go free, and that you break every yoke? Is it not to share your bread with the hungry, and that you bring to your house the poor who are cast out; when you see the naked, that you cover him, and not hide yourself from your own flesh?"[36] Jesus, in Matthew 25, tells of His coming in glory when He will sit on His throne and separate the sheep from the goats. To the sheep (the true worshipers) He says, "Come, you blessed of My Father; inherit the kingdom prepared for you from the foundation of the world: for I was hungry and you gave Me food; I was thirsty and you gave Me drink; I was a stranger and you took Me in; I was naked and you clothed Me; I was sick and you visited Me; I was in prison and you came to Me. . . . Assuredly, I say to you, inasmuch as you did it to one of the least of these My brethren, you did it to Me."[37]

We worship God by showing concern for those most in need. "Whoever receives one little child like this in My name receives Me."[38] James, the half brother of Jesus, says, "Pure and undefiled religion before God and the Father is this: to visit orphans and widows in their trouble, and to keep oneself unspotted from the world."[39] John makes clear that we must love and worship God in more than words. "Whoever has this world's goods, and sees his brother in need, and shuts up his heart from him, how does the love of God abide in him? My little children, let us not love in word or in tongue, but in deed and in truth."[40] The love we express to needy mankind is certainly a measure of love to God.

Medical Missionary Work

Beloved, let us love one another, for love is of God; and everyone who loves is born of God and knows God. He who does not love, does not know God, for God is (agape) love . . . and he who abides in love abides in God, and God in him. . . . And this commandment we have from Him: that he who loves God must love his brother also.[41]

This is stated even more strongly elsewhere:

By this we know love, because He laid down His life for us. And we also ought to lay down our lives for the brethren.[42]

This is the practical gospel—not just in word, but in practice.

Medical missionary work, as I use the term, is pure *agape* love—serving others, expecting nothing in return. While it includes unselfish medical care to others, it is not limited to what health professionals can do. It is very significant that when the King in Matthew 25 invites the righteous, because of their good deeds, "to inherit the kingdom prepared for you," their response is, "Lord, when did we see you hungry and feed You, or thirsty and give you drink? When did we see You a stranger and take You in, or naked and clothe You? Or when did we see you sick, or in prison, and come to You?"[43] They are so filled with agape love that they do not have to try to do good; they just do what comes naturally, with no thought of earning a reward or gaining merit. This is a picture of pure love—God's *agape* love.

God is waiting for this representation of His character to be revealed in our sinful world. Until a loving God in all His beauty is revealed by His children on earth, how can sinful human beings know what God is like? Paul considers "that the sufferings of this present time are not worthy to be compared with the glory which shall be revealed in us" when we show forth His love in all its beauty. "For the earnest expectation of the creation eagerly waits for the revealing of the sons of God."[44] "Beloved, now we are children of God, and it has not yet been revealed what we shall be, but we know that when He is revealed [through His human children], we shall be like Him, for we shall see Him as He is."[45]

The pure love of God as demonstrated by His human children will be "a spectacle to the world, both to angels and to men."[46] God designs that each of His children be actors in the last stage play of this world's history. The final act before "the curtain drops" is dependent on our ability, by God's grace, to love our fellow needy humans as much as God loves us. When this love is revealed in its beauty and purity, then will every person in the audience (the whole world) make their final informed choice to serve God or Satan. The world doesn't know God because it hasn't yet seen His love in us, His actors in the last drama.

When understood in these terms, medical missionary work takes a priority position. It is more than just a public relations effort of the church or an entering wedge. It is *the* key to unlocking the hearts of humans. God's unselfish love is incomprehensible to the selfish heart, but this work is designed to help God's Spirit touch sinful hearts.

This medical missionary work does not require medical training or high educational qualifications. It is much more than the selling of health services. All Christians should be doing this work. Romans 12 begins significantly with an admonition for each "not to think more highly than he ought to think, but to think soberly, as God has dealt to each one a measure of faith."[47] It then describes special gifts that have been given to some and describes how they are to be used.[48] Also in this chapter is perhaps the simplest definition of medical missionary work in the entire Bible:

Be kindly affectionate to one another with brotherly love, in honor giving preference to one another. . . . Rejoice with those who rejoice, and weep with those who weep.[49]

Empathizing with others requires not medical qualifications, but just love. The chapter ends by encouraging us "to live peaceably with all men. . . . If your enemy hungers, feed him; if he thirsts, give him a drink; for in so doing you will heap coals of fire on his head. Do not be overcome of evil, but overcome evil with good."[50] This is practical counsel which can be lived only by faith in God.

Many are surprised to hear that medical missionary work should be done by all, not just doctors, nurses, and other health professionals. However, Scripture is clear: in none of the Bible's descriptions of medical missionary work—Isaiah 58, Matthew 25, James 1, or 1 John 3—is healing mentioned. It speaks only of "visiting" the sick and "visiting" orphans and widows. God puts up no barriers to the expression of His love through us. He does not expect us all to be health professionals.

While medical missionary work is unselfish service to others, it results in tremendous blessing to the medical missionary himself. To the one who truly worships through service, this promise is given:

> Your light shall break forth like the morning, your *healing* shall spring forth speedily, and your righteousness shall go before you; the glory of the Lord shall be your rear guard. Then you shall call, and the Lord will answer; you shall cry, and He will say, 'Here I am. . . .' Then your light shall dawn in the darkness, and your darkness shall be as the noonday. The Lord will guide you continually, and satisfy your soul in drought, and *strengthen your bones*; you shall be like a watered garden, and like a spring of water, whose waters do not fail.[51]

God provides wonderful blessings for those who unselfishly minister to others.

People who feel alone and useless have three to five times the death rate of those who have a sense of community and feel useful to others.[52] Doing good for others seems to stimulate the parasympathetic nervous system. This calms our bodies and counteracts the sympathetic nervous system, which is stimulated by stress.

Healing

There is, of course, a place for healing in God's church today. Jesus set an example, and the Biblical record seems clear that Jesus spent more time healing than preaching. Everywhere He went, He healed. Sometimes people were healed "according to their faith,"[53] and once He told a newly healed man to "sin no more, lest a worse thing come upon you."[54] At other times it appears He healed all who came to Him. "His fame went throughout all Syria; and they brought to Him all sick people who were afflicted with various diseases and torments, and those who were demon possessed, epileptics, and paralytics; and He healed them."[55] In most cases the record indicates that Jesus healed without preconditions. His life exhibited unconditional love.

When Jesus sent out His disciples for their field experience, "He gave them power over unclean spirits, to cast them out, and to heal all kinds of sickness and all kinds of disease."[56] His commanded, "Heal the sick, cleanse the lepers, raise the dead, cast out demons. Freely you have received, freely give."[57] God expected His disciples to use whatever He had given them and to share it with others. The same is expected of us. Those who have been given the gift of healing must use it.[58]

Jesus explicitly promised His disciples (and us) that "He who believes in Me, the works that I do he will do also; and greater works than these he will do, because I go to My Father. . . . And I will pray the Father and He will give you another Helper, that He may abide with you forever. . . . He who has My commandments and keeps them, it is he who loves Me. And he who loves Me will be loved by My Father, and I will love him and manifest myself to him."[59] Without question, the power is available for Christ's disciples today to do all that He did and even "greater works."

Why did Jesus heal and perform miracles? At least for three reasons:

- To show His and God's love. His heart of love "was moved with compassion" for the multitudes in need.[60]

- To prove His divinity. "That you may know that the Son of Man has power on earth to forgive sins," He said to the paralytic, "Arise, take up your bed. . . ."[61] Another time Jesus said, "though you do not believe Me, believe the works, that you may know and believe that the Father is in Me, and I in Him."[62]

- To demonstrate what man could become with God's help. Man had sunk so low at the time of His first advent that Jesus felt it necessary to miraculously heal in order to show what it really means to be restored in God's image—to be whole and in good health. Because His time in His public ministry was short, He had to demonstrate health quickly. He did not have enough time to allow the natural process of restoration to occur. Christ also sought to demonstrate not just ordinary life, but "life more abundant."[63]

The needs we face today are much different than what Jesus faced. Could this mean that God's plan for His healing ministry is different today than when Jesus walked on earth?

The seventy returned from their mission rejoicing and saying,"Lord, even the demons are subject to us in Your name."[64] Christ's thought-provoking response was this: "Do not rejoice in this, that the spirits are subject to you, but rather rejoice because your names are written in heaven."[65] In effect, Jesus said miracles are less important than whether you are living a life that assures your name is written in the Book of Life. This, to me, strongly infers that miracles by Christ's disciples now are less important than in Christ's time.

Following are some conditions that are different now than when Christ was on earth. If true, these dictate a different role for healing ministries.

1. Christ proved His divinity by His life on earth, by His miracles, and especially by His death and resurrection. We no longer have to carry the burden of that proof. Jesus completed the proof of His divinity. We introduce the Biblical, historical Christ, and invite the Holy Spirit to confirm His divinity in hearts that are open to Him.

2. Miracles will be a special effort of the Devil in the last days. "For false christs and false prophets will rise and show great signs and wonders to deceive, if possible, even the elect."[66] Jesus forewarned us not to be deceived by false miracles. He said, "Many will say to Me in that day, 'Lord, Lord, have we not prophesied in Your name and done many wonders in Your name?' And then I will declare to them, 'I never knew you; depart from Me, you who practice lawlessness.'"[67] Two tests are given to distinguish false miracle workers from the true: (1) "To the law and to the testimony! If they do not speak according to this word, it is because there is no light in them."[68] (2) "Beware of false prophets . . . by their fruits you will know them."[69]

3. God urgently desires to prepare a people for His soon coming. The preparation of Israel for the Promised Land is an example of how He works. The first promise to Israel after the triumphal crossing of the Red Sea was this: "If you diligently heed the voice of the Lord your God and do what is right in His sight, give ear to His commandments and keep all His statutes, I will put none of the diseases on you which I have brought on the Egyptians. For I am the Lord who heals you."[70] Their preparation included dietary reform and a system of hygiene based on God's laws of health. The New Testament outlines the preparation necessary for Christ's second coming: "For the grace of God that brings salvation has appeared to all men, teaching us that, denying ungodliness and worldly lusts, *we should live soberly, righteously, and godly* in the present age, looking for the blessed hope and glorious appearing of our great God and Savior Jesus Christ, who gave himself for us, that He might redeem us from every lawless deed and purify for Himself His own special people, zealous for good works."[71] Satan says it is impossible to live a godly life in this world, while Satan himself does all he can to make it difficult. Only with the help of God can we live holy, sanctified lives in preparation for His advent. To do so is our special challenge in these last days, and God's help is clearly promised. "Now may the God of peace

Himself sanctify you completely; and may your whole spirit, soul, and *body be preserved blameless* at the coming of our Lord Jesus Christ. He who calls you is faithful, *who also will do it.*"[72]

4. A priority today is to prepare a people who understand that following God's way leads to life and health and builds character, while following Satan's way leads to disease and death. Rather than provide miraculous healing, God has given His people extra time to go through the process of restoration that they might (a) fully comprehend the beauty of His law and (b) build characters for eternity. Paul recognized the need of this when he said, "I discipline my body and bring it into subjection, lest, when I have preached to others, I myself should become disqualified."[73] In another place he admonishes us to "work out your own salvation with fear and trembling; for it is God who works in you both to will and to do for His good pleasure."[74] Again he says, "I can do all things through Christ who strengthens me."[75] By understanding God's purposes and His way, we will eventually sing with David, "I delight to do Your will, O my God, and Your law is within my heart."[76] God's laws, physical and moral, are gifts that teach us how to do His will.

In the last days of earth's history, health and healing have a special role in helping people build character and prepare for heaven. It is our privilege to show, through faith in God and by His help, what sanctified living is. This is best revealed in our everyday living.

Meditation

True worship also includes prayer and meditation. Recently, meditation has become immensely popular in medical circles. Evidence shows that it provides remarkable physical and psychological benefits. Physicians use it to increase relaxation, lower blood pressure, decrease pain, reduce secretion of stress hormones, and decrease the amount of excess stomach acid in people with gastrointestinal problems. Patients, through meditation, tend to view themselves as healthier, better able to handle stressful situations, and more in control of their lives.[77]

Some define meditation as "mindfulness—paying purposeful attention, becoming fully aware of the present moment."[78] Ornish suggests that meditation is "the art of paying attention," and says it is particularly useful for controlling eating habits. Meals which begin with a prayer of gratitude and thankfulness tend to be eaten more peacefully, with joy and awareness. "Eating with awareness" can help one enjoy meals more fully, noticing how food affects the body. For instance, after a rich, fatty meal, one feels tired and sluggish; after eating low-fat starchy foods, one feels more energetic, and food is digested more effectively.[79]

Meditation provides several benefits:

- Powers of concentration increase.
- Awareness of surroundings increases.
- Awareness of the inner body increases; it becomes easier to notice the effects of food and recognize when enough has been eaten.
- The mind becomes quieter and more peaceful; sleep comes easier and deeper.
- A person's picture of self becomes clearer and less distorted.
- Worries about the past and future decrease; it becomes easier to live in the present.
- A person gains food for the soul and peace for the spirit.[80]

Meditation has a clear Biblical background, but recently Eastern religions have taken it over to an extent that many Christians are now afraid of it. True, it can be used for the physical benefits alone and not in worship of God. Christian meditation needs to be differentiated from that of Eastern religions. Eastern meditation emphasizes emptying the mind, losing individuality, and merging with the "Cosmic Mind." The final goal is detachment—escaping from the miserable wheel of existence into Nirvana (nothingness). Zen and Yoga are popular forms of Eastern meditation and worship.

Transcendental Meditation (TM), with its Buddhist roots, is a modern aberration designed for the secularist—a method of controlling the brain waves in order to improve physiological and emotional well-being. The secular person, seeking to live in a purely physical universe, uses TM to obtain the physiological benefits of a consistent alpha brain-wave pattern. But seeking only physical benefits is a selfish approach to meditation.

Christian meditation is an effort to open the mind to God's presence. One detaches from the confusion around in order to obtain a richer attachment to God. All are called to enter into the living presence of God for themselves, but it is serious and awesome work to invite God, through His Spirit, to literally enter our minds.

The discipline of meditation must be learned. Following are some practical hints and exercises for beginners. These are not rules, but just a few windows to the inner world where Christ loves to dwell.

- Set aside some time each day for contemplative prayer and meditation. Ideally, however, it must become a way of life. "Pray without ceasing,"[81] Paul urges. Lives constantly harassed and fragmented by external affairs are not prepared for meditation. We will be better prepared for meditation if we learn to balance and live at peace all day long.

- Choose a place for meditation. It should be quiet and free from interruptions. Stay away from the telephone. Natural surroundings are best.

- You can pray and meditate any time, anywhere, and in any position. No single posture is required. Find the most comfortable and least distracting position for you, keeping in mind that a posture of peace and relaxation has a tendency to calm inner turmoil. (Inner tension is almost always signaled by body language. For instance, a person vigorously chewing gum shows they are not relaxed.) For most people, sitting quietly in a straight chair with both feet flat on the floor is very conducive to meditation. Slouching indicates inattention, and crossing the legs restricts circulation. You may want to close your eyes to help remove distractions and center your attention on Christ. Regardless of how it is done, the aim is to center the attention of the body, emotions, mind, and spirit upon the "knowledge of the glory of God in the face of Jesus Christ."[82]

- Probably the inner world of meditation is most easily entered through the door of imagination. Rare individuals may be able to contemplate a blank void, but most need to have their thoughts rooted in the senses. Jesus taught this way, using parables that constantly appealed to the imagination and senses. Ignatius of Loyola, in his *Spiritual Exercises,* encouraged visualization of the Gospel stories. We should try to utilize all five senses as we imagine Gospel events. Smell the sea. Hear the water lapping along the shore. See the crowd. Feel the sun on your head and the hunger in your stomach. Taste the salt in the air. Touch the hem of His garment.

- We should progress as fast as possible in our spiritual life, but we must begin somewhere. For most, it works best to start with five or ten minutes a day. The first effort is to learn to **center down**—to become quiet, to enter into recreating silence, to allow the fragmentation of our minds to become centered on the object of meditation. Turn all your concerns and worries over to the Lord and spend this precious time in silence. Do not ask for anything. Allow the Lord to commune with your spirit, to love you. If impressions or directions come, fine; if not, fine.

- After gaining some proficiency in centering down, add five or ten minutes to meditate on an aspect of God's creation. It may be a tree, a plant, a bird, a leaf, an insect, some part of the human body, or anything else you choose to prayerfully ponder. God wants to show us something of His glory in His creation. "For since the creation of the world His invisible attributes are clearly seen, being understood by the things that are made, even His eternal power and Godhead, so that they are without excuse."[83]

- Having learned through these exercises, turn to Scripture. The Word of God should be the reference point by which all other meditations are kept in perspective. Meditation involves internalizing and personalizing specific passages of Scripture. The written Word becomes a living message addressed to each one personally. By entering into a Bible story, not as a passive observer but as an active participant, one can actually encounter the living Christ. It becomes more than an exercise of imagination; it is a genuine confrontation. Jesus Christ is actually with you by His Spirit! This is not the time for technical word studies or even to gather material to share with others. This is the time to receive with humble heart the Word personally addressed to you. Kneeling is often the best posture for this encounter with our Lord. The words God puts in your heart may be words you need to ponder for days on end, following the example of Mary, who "kept all these things and pondered them in her heart."[84] You will want to live with and experience your chosen Scripture as a special guide for that day.

- "Rest in the Lord, and wait patiently for Him."[85] Listen quietly in your silent meditation, anticipating the unanticipated. Note carefully any instruction given. With time and experience you will learn to distinguish between mere human thoughts and the voice of the Holy Spirit, which moves inwardly upon the heart, usually through words of Scripture. Do not be surprised if the instruction is terribly practical and not at all what you thought of as "spiritual." Do not be disappointed if no word comes; like good friends, you and God are silently enjoying the each other's company. Don't be discouraged if your meditations hold little meaning for you in the beginning. Remember, you are learning an art for which you have received no training. Our culture discourages—or at least does nothing to develop—these skills. Take heart. The effort will be immensely worthwhile.

- At the end of each meditation, close with a genuine expression of thanksgiving to God. Return to the outside world with new life from on high.[86]

Relationship of Meditation to the Sabbath

Harvey Cox, a Harvard Divinity School professor, speaks of the similarity between Christian meditation and Sabbath keeping. He points out that Christianity has its own contemplative tradition. Despite His busy life, Jesus often took time to withdraw and be alone. Today, however, most Christian churches have failed to teach people how to pray and meditate. Few know spiritual discipline at all. Christians, rather than adapting Buddhist or Eastern forms, need to uncover the roots of meditation in Biblical tradition. A knowledge of Jewish background is especially helpful.

Professor Cox gained his insights when invited to spend a Sabbath with a rabbi in Colorado. Here he describes this experience:

A rabbi who lives in a small town near Boulder invited me to join him and his tiny congregation in celebrating the weekly Sabbath, not just the religious service that took place in his backyard, but a genuine, old-fashioned *Shabbat*, a whole day of doing very little, enjoying the creation as it is, appreciating the world rather than fixing it up. I accepted the invitation and joined in a relaxed Sabbath, which lasted, as tradition dictates, from Friday sundown until sundown on Saturday. During those luminous hours, as we talked quietly, slept, ate, repeated the ancient Hebrew prayers, and savored just being, rather than doing, it occurred to me that meditation is in essence a kind of miniature Sabbath. . . .

The word for Sabbath in Hebrew comes from a root meaning "to desist." Sabbath originally meant a time that was designated for ceasing all activity and simply acknowledging the goodness of creation. . . . [In the Hebrew tradition] it represents the Israelites' recognition that although human beings can catch a glimpse of the pure realm of unity and innocence, they also live in the fractured world of division, greed, and sorrow. Sabbath is Israel's ingenious attempt to live both in history and beyond it, both in time and eternity. . . .

At first reading, the suggestion that God "rested" after the toil of creation— the image of a craftsman sitting down and wiping his brow—sounds quaintly anthropomorphic. The word "rest" literally means "to catch one's breath". . . . The first thing to notice about God's activity on the Sabbath is that it focuses on breathing. We all stop to draw breath after we have been exerting ourselves, and the passage may mean no more than this. But to depict God himself as one who ceases work and does nothing but breathe could suggest a deeper and older stratum of spiritual consciousness that lies behind the passage itself. Breath is a source of renewal, and God, like human beings, returns periodically to the source. . . .

The spirit of Sabbath is a Biblical equivalent of meditation. . . . It is a particular form of consciousness, a way of thinking called "mindfulness". . . . Sabbath excludes manipulative ways of thinking about the world. Abraham Heschel repeats a story that exemplifies this point well.

A certain rabbi, it seems, who was renowned for his wisdom and piety, and especially for his zeal in keeping Sabbath, once took a leisurely walk in his garden on the Sabbath day—an activity that even the severest interpreters allowed. Strolling among the fruit trees, the rabbi noticed that one of the apple trees badly needed pruning. Recognizing that, of course, such a thing could not be done on the seventh day, the rabbi nonetheless made a mental note to himself that he would see to the pruning early the next week. The Sabbath passed. But when the rabbi went out to the tree a few days later with ladder and clippers, he found it shriveled and life-less. God had destroyed the apple tree to teach the rabbi that even *thinking* about work on the Sabbath is a violation of the commandment and of the true spirit of the Holy Day.

When we plan to prune a tree, we perceive it differently from when we are simply aware of it, allowing it—for the moment at least—simply to be as it is. . . . This "mindfulness" or "bare awareness" is strengthened by the practice of meditation. It is being aware, fully aware, of the apple tree, but having no judgments, plans, or prospects for it. . . .

When the sun goes down and the lamps begin to flicker on Friday evening, a kind of magic touches the (Hebrew) world. Special cakes have been baked and now the sacred candles are lighted. Sabbath is eternity in time, as Abraham Heschel says; it is a cathedral made not with stones and glass but with hours and minutes. It is a sacred symbol that no one can tear down or destroy. It comes every week, inviting human beings not to strive and succeed, not even to pray very much, but to taste and know that God is good, that the earth and the flesh are there to be shared and enjoyed. . . .

Sabbath is the key to a Biblical understanding of meditation. True medi-tation does not take the place of the gathered congregation, of celebrating and breaking bread. But it can restore the Sabbath insight that, despite all the things that *must* be done in the world—to feed and liberate and heal—even God occasionally pauses to draw breath. Sabbath is a reminder that there will again be a time, as there once was a time, when toil and pain will cease, when play and song and just sitting will fill out the hours and days, when we will no longer require the rhythm of work and repose because there will be no real difference between them. Sabbath reminds us that that day will come, but it also reminds us that that day is not yet here. We need both reminders. . . .

The person whose vision of the world is derived from Biblical faith rather than from the wisdom of the Orient can incorporate meditation as a part of a daily dialectic of withdrawal and involvement, of clarification and action. . . . We may discover that meditation can restore a lost treasure, the "Fourth Commandment." It may be tarnished and twisted out of shape, but it still belongs to us: and as creatures who must live amid the contra-dictions and dislocations of history, the mini-Sabbath of meditation can be the gift of life itself.[87]

Meditation and the Sabbath *do* complement one another. It is no accident that Isaiah connects the true worship of unselfish ministry—what I call medical missionary work—with building "old waste places," raising "the foundation of many generations," and calling "the Sabbath a delight."[88]

Summary: True Worship

The third angel warns against false worship and its terrible consequences. True worship, through prayer and meditation, through care of our bodies as the temple of God's Spirit, and through demonstrating God's *agape* love to the most needy in this world, brings healing, health, and a special relationship with God. Good thinking, as a part of true worship, also brings its rewards:

For as he thinks in his heart, so is he.[89]

Finally, brethren, whatever things are true, whatever things are noble, whatever things are just, whatever things are pure, whatever things are lovely, whatever things are of good report, if there is an virtue and there is anything praiseworthy—meditate on these things.[90]

Only the true worshiper receives this invitation from the King:

Come, you blessed of My Father, inherit the kingdom prepared for you from the foundation of the world.[91]

Isaiah 58 assures the true worshiper, "The Lord will guide you continually, and satisfy your soul in drought, and strengthen your bones." Remember that these same bones supply the white blood cells that make up the immune system.

You shall be like a watered garden and like a spring of water whose waters do not fail. Those from among you shall build the old waste places; you shall raise up the foundations of many generations; and you shall be called the Repairer of the Breach, the Restorer of Streets to Dwell In.[92]

God's true worshipers are the ones who will prepare the way for His coming. When His love is powerfully revealed to the world, all people will be able to make a final choice for or against Him. Those who are open to His Spirit will take their stand as His children. This cannot be accomplished by argument or preaching, but by a perfect demonstration of God's love in human hearts.

The great medical missionary chapter of the Bible, Isaiah 58, ends with the reassurance that true medical missionaries "call the Sabbath a delight."[93] True worshipers are given this promise:

Then you shall delight yourself in the Lord; and I will cause you to ride on the high hills of the earth, and feed you with the heritage of Jacob your father. The mouth of the Lord has spoken.[94]

Those who wait on the Lord (in meditation), shall renew their strength;

they shall mount up with wings like eagles, they shall run and not be weary, they shall walk and not faint.[95]

Prayer

Dear God, we praise You for Your wonderful plan to overcome the beast and his image. We raise our hearts in adoration to You, for You loved us and died for us while we were still sinners. We ask Your Spirit to lead us into deeper fellowship with You. Give us wisdom that we may know Your love and reveal it fully to those in greatest need. May the words of our mouths and the meditation of our hearts be acceptable in Your sight. Amen.

---

[1] Galatians 6:7, 8.
[2] Romans 6:23.
[3] Genesis 2:16, 17.
[4] Genesis 3:4.
[5] John 11:11-14.
[6] Ecclesiastes 9:5.
[7] 1 Timothy 6:16.
[8] Genesis 2:7.
[9] 1 Corinthians 15:51-54.
[10] Revelation 14:11.
[11] Malachi 4:1-3.
[12] Psalms 37:10, 20, and 36.
[13] 2 Peter 3:12, 13; Revelation 21:1, 2.
[14] Jude 7.
[15] Mark 9:43, 45.
[16] Jeremiah 17:27.
[17] Obadiah 8:16.
[18] Isaiah 47:14.
[19] 2 Peter 3:9.
[20] Jonah 3:10.
[21] Ephesians 2:4.
[22] 1 Peter 3:19; Genesis 6.
[23] Revelation 14:9.
[24] *Merriam-Webster's Collegiate Dictionary* (Merriam-Webster, 10th ed., 1993).
[25] 1 Thessalonians 5:17.
[26] Philippians 4:6.
[27] Psalm 19:14.
[28] 1 Timothy 4:5.
[29] Psalm 119:11, 105.
[30] Hebrews 4:12.
[31] 1 Corinthians 6:19, 20.
[32] Revelation 14:7.
[33] Romans 12:1.
[34] Philippians 4:13.

[35] Romans 12:2.
[36] Isaiah 58:6, 7.
[37] Matthew 25:31-40.
[38] Matthew 18:5.
[39] James 1:27.
[40] 1 John 3:18.
[41] 1 John 4:7, 8, 16, and 21.
[42] 1 John 3:16.
[43] Matthew 25:37-39.
[44] Romans 8:18, 19.
[45] 1 John 3:2.
[46] 1 Corinthians 4:9.
[47] Romans 12:3.
[48] Romans 12:4-8.
[49] Romans 12:10, 15, and 16.
[50] Romans 12:18-21.
[51] Isaiah 58:8-11.
[52] Dean Ornish, MD, "Isolation . . . and Your Heart," *Bottom Line Personal* 15 July 1992: 11-13.
[53] For example, Luke 8:48; 17:19; 18:42.
[54] John 5:14.
[55] Matthew 4:24.
[56] Matthew 10:1.
[57] Matthew 10:8.
[58] 1 Corinthians 12:9.
[59] John 14:12, 16, and 21.
[60] Matthew 9:36.
[61] Matthew 9:6.
[62] John 10:38.
[63] John 10:10.
[64] Luke 10:17.
[65] Luke 10:20.
[66] Matthew 24:24.
[67] Matthew 7:22, 23.
[68] Isaiah 8:20.
[69] Matthew 7:15-20.
[70] Exodus 15:26.
[71] Titus 2:11-14.
[72] 1 Thessalonians 5:23, 24.
[73] 1 Corinthians 9:27.
[74] Philippians 2:12, 13.
[75] Colossians 4:13.
[76] Psalm 40:8.
[77] Jon Kabat-Zinn, PhD, "Mindfulness Meditation . . . to Improve Your Life," *Bottom Line Personal* 21 Feb. 1991: 11.
[78] Ibid.
[79] Dean Ornish, MD, *Eat More, Weigh Less* (Harper Perrenial, 1993) 69-73.
[80] Ibid, 74, 75.
[81] 1 Thessalonians 5:17.

82 2 Corinthians 4:6.

83 Romans 1:20.

84 Luke 2:19.

85 Psalm 37:7.

86 Condensed and adapted from Richard J. Foster, "The Discipline of Meditation," *Celebration of Discipline: The Path to Spiritual Growth* (Harper & Row, 1978).

87 Harvey Cox, "Meditation and Sabbath," *Harvard Magazine* Sept.-Oct. 1977: 39-43 and 68. This article was excerpted from Cox's book *Turning East: the Promise and Peril of New Orientalism* (Simon and Schuster, 1977).

88 Isaiah 58:12, 13.

89 Proverbs 23:7.

90 Philippians 4:8.

91 Matthew 25:34.

92 Isaiah 58:11, 12.

93 Isaiah 58:13.

94 Isaiah 58:14.

95 Isaiah 40:31.

CHAPTER TEN

No Rest
Day or Night

AND THEY HAVE NO REST DAY OR NIGHT, WHO WORSHIP THE BEAST AND HIS IMAGE, AND WHOEVER RECEIVES THE MARK OF HIS NAME. REVELATION 14:11

After describing the final judgment on those who "worship the beast and his image," the third angel adds a postscript. "And they have no rest day or night, who worship the beast and his image, and whoever receives the mark of his name."[1] Not only do those who worship the beast and his image have a terrible end, but while living "they have no rest day or night." How can one rest when the mind is filled with fear, guilt, and anxiety? Negative thoughts disturb rest and decrease the immune system's ability to resist disease. Let's take a deeper look at the relationship between negative thoughts and health.

Stress and Health

Stress ranked as the number one health concern in a recent survey of executives polled by *Business & Health*.[2] A recent *U. S. News & World Report* cover story entitled "Stressed Out?" depicted a man's face on a steaming tea kettle. The article reported that seven of 10 respondents said they felt stress at some point during a typical workday—30 percent said they experienced a lot of stress; 40 percent reported feeling some. Forty-three percent of U.S. adults suffer noticeable physical and emotional symptoms of burnout. Somewhere between 75 and 90 percent of all doctor office visits stem from stress.[3] Anxiety disorders are the most prevalent of all mental illnesses; however, depression ranks a close second and is increasing around the world.

Simply defined, stress is the way the body reacts, physically and emotionally, to change. (It is frequently referred to in scientific literature as "what happens when perceived threats chronically activate the body's 'fight or flight' response."[4]) Stress works positively when it helps one to concentrate, perform, and reach peak efficiency mentally or physically. Positive stress is followed by a relaxation response that allows body and mind to recover and prepare for next challenge. Negative stress, on the other hand, occurs when stimulation continues indefinitely without time to relax and recover. Negative stress is what most people mean when they speak of "stress," and this problem has been linked to multiple physical ailments.[5]

Physiological reactions to stress include the body's effort to prepare for **fight or flight**. For a short term this can give the body an advantage, but if a person feels overwhelmed rather than challenged, stress becomes a burden. It causes depression and insomnia, strains the heart and nervous system, and poses a long-term danger to the entire body. Stress-related disorders include angina, palpitations of the heart, elevated blood cholesterol levels, high blood pressure, heart attacks and strokes, asthma, auto-immune diseases, painful menstruation, indigestion, peptic ulcer, colitis, constipation, eczema, tension headaches, and psychosis. By depressing the immune system, stress makes people more vulnerable to cancer, infections, and other disorders.

Negative stress initially produces an **alarm reaction**. Blood pressure increases; heart rate increases; blood flow to muscles increases; blood flow to skin and kidneys decreases; respiration rate increases; gastrointestinal activity decreases; blood sugar, blood fats, and blood cholesterol increase, as does blood coagulation; muscle strength and mental activity increase. A body cannot maintain such a state for a prolonged period without sustaining functional or structural damage. Therefore, the body begins to adapt to the situation within a few hours. During prolonged stress, blood pressure drops but still stays above normal; the heart slows but still beats fifteen times a minute faster than normal; the stomach works, but at a reduced level which interferes with good digestion.

One type of stress is caused by disharmonic music. The body is designed to be in harmony with itself, nature, and God. Many physiological functions have their own cycles and rhythms—e.g. the heart beat, respiratory rate, and the day/night cycle. The stress of disharmonic music disrupts these rhythms; it has been associated with deviant behaviors such as introversion, despondency and depression, nervousness, wild unpredictable behavior, and extreme aggression. It has been shown to cause hyperactivity, heightened mob instinct, abnormal fears, bad attitudes, lethargy or laziness, and impaired memory and learning. Disharmonic music leads to an emotional imbalance in which judgment cannot be trusted.[6]

Two doctors did a study of music and the nervous system. Mice were divided into three groups. Those in Group H were exposed to classical harmonic music; Group D listened to discordant rock music; and Group C was a control group kept in a quiet environment. After three months of constant day-and-night exposure to the music, it turned out that mice exposed to discordant sounds had more difficulties with learning and memory than those in the control group. They also incurred structural changes in their brain cells—abnormal branching and sprouting of the neurons in an effort to compensate for the stress caused by disharmonic rhythms.

The amount of messenger RNA was also different between Group D and C. The study group mice showed deviant behavior ranging from hyperactivity and aggression to lethargy and inattentiveness. Differences between the control group and mice exposed to classical music were few.[7]

There appears to be no middle road with music. It either enhances the Creator's design and nature's pull toward optimum (harmonic) balance, or it interferes with that balance. It either uplifts or degrades physiologic and psychologic functions.

Activities or actions which cause stress can be viewed in various ways. Holmes and Rahe have established a **stress scale** that considers death of a spouse as 100 and other stressors are comparatively less. On their scale, a jail term is 63; marriage, 50; a mortgage debt over $10,000, 31; an outstanding personal achievement, 28; and a vacation, 13.[8] Note that stressors are not necessarily bad events. Even notable achievements and vacations tend to upset an individual's equilibrium and require adaptation.

All stress is individualized. It is not so much an activity as a personal reaction to change or a perceived threat. It is the individual's response that really counts, and poor coping can be modified. **Coping** is a learned skill that will be addressed later in this chapter.

The Immune System

The immune system is the body's vital mechanism for fighting disease. It protects the body from harmful materials and organisms that cause disease. Cells of the immune system (white blood cells) circulate throughout the body. Although there are different kinds of white blood cells, the lymphocytes are especially important for immunity. The two major types both arise from precursors in the bone marrow—(1) the B lymphocytes develop in the liver and spleen and produce antibodies, and (2) the T lymphocytes—the phagocytes—develop in the thymus and provide cellular immunity by directly attacking and devouring invaders.

Although related closely to both the nervous and hormonal systems, the organs of the immune system are positioned throughout the body. They are called lymphoid organs because they are home to the lymphocytes. Lymphocytes travel through the body either by way of the blood vessels or by their own lymph-carrying vessels. Small, bean-shaped lymph nodes are laced along the lymphatic vessels and clustered together in the neck, armpits, abdomen, and groin. The thymus and spleen are special organs in which immune cells gather to work. Clumps of lymphoid tissue are also found in other parts of the body, especially in the digestive tract lining and in the airways and lungs—potential gateways to the body. These tissue clumps include the tonsils, adenoids, and appendix—organs which until recently were often surgically removed by doctors who did not realize their importance in the immune system.[9]

Most of us have experienced the connection between stress and getting sick. In my case, colds are usually preceded by such stressors as fatigue, discouragement, and/or mild depression. Stress, originating in the mind, induces the hypothalamus and pituitary to produce steroid hormones, which suppress cellular immunity.[10]

Connections between negative psychological states (such as anxiety and depression) and the immune system have been explored. The results suggest that depressed and anxious moods are associated with decreases in lymphocyte proliferation and natural killer cell activity. In addition, there are changes in the number of white blood cells and the quantity of antibody circulating in the blood. The greater the level of anxiety, the less antibody is produced after exposure to a potentially harmful substance. The longer the stress, the greater the decrease in white blood cells.

Stress is also associated with behaviors that affect the immune system. Stressed people tend to sleep less, exercise less, have poorer diets, smoke more, and use alcohol and other drugs more often. These factors decrease the immune system's ability to fight disease, although further research is needed to better clarify these relationships.[11] For now, it is clear that prolonged stress directly and indirectly harms the immune system and predisposes the hyper-stressed body to disease.

Negative Emotions

Negative emotions such as anger, hate, frustration, discontentment, fear, anxiety, distrust, and depression occur frequently as reactions to stress. These emotions intensify the negative effects of stress on the immune system. The World Health Organization (WHO) points out that because

> self-interest is such a strong force, we continue to defend ourselves and preserve our selfish interests. . . . The decline in virtue—defined as control of passions and emotions, and directing them along beneficial channels for the common good rather than self-interest—has caused the destruction of peace in individuals, families, communities, countries and the whole world.[12]

The relationship between personality types and heart attacks was much publicized in the 1950s. Cardiologists Meyer Friedman and Ray Rosenman discovered that impatient Type A people—those who walked and ate quickly, interrupted others, and drove themselves relentlessly—were more likely to suffer heart problems than their calmer Type B peers—those who were more relaxed, controlled, and purposeful. Anxious, tense Type A people are generally successful in business and the professions. Dr. R. Williams of Duke University Medical Center has tried to determine what factor is most closely associated with their heart disease. He suggests that "*cynicism*, better than any other single word, captures the toxic element in the Type A personality." He goes on to say that "those who expect the worst from the world around them might find themselves leaving it sooner "—with a heart attack.

In Williams' study, those who had high levels of hostility, as measured on the MMPI (Minnesota Multiphasic Personality Inventory), were 50 percent more likely to have clogged coronary arteries than those who scored low. A study was done on 255 physicians who were administered the MMPI during their residency training. Twenty-five years later, those with high hostility scores had five times more heart disease than those who scored below the median. A similar study of lawyers found that of those who scored in the top quarter for hostility, one in five was dead by age 50. Of those in the lowest quarter, only one in 25 had died.[13]

More recently a Type C personality has been described—people who are super nice, happy, and in control. However, these people tend to be rigid, conforming individuals who lack satisfactory emotional outlets. They may bottle up anger and other strong emotions. They also tend to be depressed, feeling hopeless and helpless in the face of stress. Such people seem especially susceptible to cancer.[14] In a 17-year study of 2,000 middle-aged men, depression was associated with twice the risk of death from cancer when compared with non-depressed men.[15]

A study by Dr. Murray Mittleman of Harvard Medical School reported in 1994 on the role of acute anger in contrast to chronic hostility. His study suggests the average risk of heart attack more than doubles in the two hours following an outburst of moderate or greater anger. Anger increases the heart rate and blood pressure, which may damage plaques inside the coronary arteries, thus leading to heart attacks.[16]

Can or should we get rid of anger? No. As long as the devil is causing injustice in the world, there is a place for righteous indignation. However, while there may be a place for anger, there is clearly no place for angry action. Apostle Paul warns,

> Be angry, and do not sin; do not let the sun go down on your wrath, nor give place [an opportunity] to the devil. . . . Let no corrupt word proceed out of your mouth, but what is good for necessary edification, that it may impart grace to the hearers. . . . Let all bitterness, wrath, anger, clamor [loud quarreling], and evil speaking be put away from you, with all malice. And be kind to one another, tenderhearted, forgiving one another, even as God in Christ forgave you.[17]

Psychologists are increasingly convinced that the harmful effects of anger are not in the anger itself. Three types of reactions should be avoided. (1) Trying to **deny or repress** anger is not good. It needs to be expressed in some way. (2) **Giving vent** to anger in words or actions, even just the gritting of teeth, is bad physiologically. (3) Perhaps the worst is the so-called permanent "**free-floating hostility**," in which a person is perpetually suspicious, wary, snappish, and forever tense.

Aron Siegman, a psychologist with the Baltimore V.A. Hospital, has done much study on anger. He says, "Give in to your anger and you become all the more angry. Resist it, and the anger seeps away." He points out that Freudian psychoanalysts view anger as physical energy which must either be expressed or repressed, but Siegman says, "an angry person who chooses to divert his attention will no longer be angry. We have a lot of evidence to show that." The person who follows Siegman's advice neither denies his rage nor gives in to it. Anger can be calmly talked out and released so that it neither festers nor explodes but gradually loses its hold.[18] Perhaps his suggestions give us a clue on how to handle many negative emotions. Fear, for example, can be recognized as providing energy to do one's best in a new situation; guilt can be seen as initiating the process of beneficial lifestyle changes.[19] We need to encourage the diversion of negative emotions to useful purposes.

The emotions you allow to hold sway in your mind profoundly influence your health. "For as he thinks in his heart, so is he."[20] Dr. Hans Selye, the author of the modern concept of stress, made this remarkable statement:

It seems to me that, among all the emotions, there is one which, more than any other, accounts for the absence or presence of stress in human relations: that is the feeling of gratitude—with its negative counterpart—the need for revenge.[21]

Similarly, another author has written:

Nothing tends more to promote health of body and of soul than does a spirit of gratitude and praise. It is a positive duty to resist melancholy, discontented thoughts and feelings—as much a duty as it is to pray.[22]

In another place she writes,

The condition of the mind affects the health to a far greater degree than many realize. Many of the diseases from which men suffer are the result of mental depression. Grief, anxiety, discontent, remorse, guilt, distrust, all tend to break down the life forces and to invite decay and death.[23]

Stress Management

Dr. Carl Thoreson of Stanford University suggests a six-stage program for coping with stress and lifestyle changes: (1) **identify the problem**—the stressor and its personal effect on you; (2) **commit to change** and build confidence that change is possible; (3) develop an **awareness of stress sources** and your response to them—what can you do differently; (4) develop a stress management **action plan**, including specific relaxation techniques and stress avoidance and/or control methods; (5) regularly and frequently **evaluate** your plan, recognizing successes or unrealistic expectations and modifying the plan appropriately; (6) maintain gains achieved by recognizing the need for **daily discipline** and permanent lifestyle changes.[24]

Dr. Timothy W. Brigham of Jefferson Medical College points out that people develop habitual ways of reacting to stress. Some of these habits (with Brigham's suggested changes) include:

Deficiency-focusing—the habit of focusing on the negative at the expense of the positive; expecting things to go wrong. To change this ask, "What's right?" Gain perspective by placing situations in their proper context. Think, for instance, "How can the obstacles I face be overcome?"

Necessitating—thinking something has to be done rather than recognizing one has a choice. If every request is interpreted as a demand, calamity is expected when one does not live up to the demands. To change this ask, "What can realistically happen if I don't do this?" or "Is there room for negotiation?"

Low skill recognition—the tendency not to recognize one's abilities and successes. Everything positive is attributed to something external—luck or another person. To change this self-defeating attitude, recognize limitations while also acknowledging one's developing skills and abilities. Look for ways to gain experience, confidence, and self-esteem.[25]

An article in the *American Journal of Preventive Medicine* finds that four factors have repeatedly emerged as successful strategies in resisting stress. These coping strategies are associated with lower incidence of physical illness, lower amounts of anxiety and depression, and increased longevity. The factors are as follows:

• Personal control. Planned, organized, self-directed activity reduces stress and subsequent illness. Those who allow others to make their decisions for them or who perceive control as external, risk greater physical and psychologic distress.

• Task involvement. Personal involvement and commitment to a task that one considers important and meaningful appears to be a powerful factor leading to better individual health.

• Lifestyle choices. Stress-resistant people are willing to change their diets and lifestyles when they recognize change can produce clearer thinking and an increased sense of well-being.

• Social supports. Relationships with others can buffer stress and provide emotional and other helpful support. Feelings of isolation are very detrimental to health.[26]

There are obviously many approaches to stress management. The lifestyle advocated in this book is designed to make one resistant to stress. The best diet for strengthening one's immune system and stress resistance is one high in starchy foods (complex carbohydrates), low in fat, and rich in antioxidant vitamins, minerals, phytochemicals, and fiber (as described in Chapter 4). It includes a balanced lifestyle with a good exercise program (as described in Chapter 6). It includes a worshipful attitude toward God as described in Chapter 9). Some additional suggestions are included here.

A body under stress experiences excessive muscle tension. This is often subtle and difficult to detect. If muscle tension continues for long periods, it causes a variety of physical problems, including tension headaches (the most common type of headache), muscle cramps, limited range of joint motion and poor flexibility, insomnia, constipation, and many other functional disorders. Relaxation exercises serve as a natural treatment for neuromuscular tension. These include (1) **deep breathing**, (2) **progressive muscular relaxation**, and (3) **stretching**.

> **Deep breathing**. Slow and shallow breathing is an automatic reaction to stress. Consciously initiated deep breathing can be done anywhere, and should be done at least three times a day, or whenever one begins to feel tense.
>
> Begin by sitting or standing (with good posture) and placing your hands firmly on your abdomen. Inhale slowly and deeply through your nose, letting your stomach expand as much as possible. When you have breathed in as much as possible, hold your breath for a few seconds, then exhale slowly through your mouth, pursing your lips as if you were going to whistle. Pursing your lips helps you to control how fast you exhale. When your lungs feel empty, begin the inhale-exhale cycle again. Repeat this cycle three or four times at each session.
>
> **Progressive muscular relaxation**. This technique can help you actually feel the difference between tension and relaxation. It can be done while sitting or lying down and takes about fifteen minutes to complete. Try it in a quiet, relaxed atmosphere. You may start with the hands, then progress to other muscles, or you may begin by moving from head to toe, tightening and relaxing the muscles in the face, shoulders, arms, hands, chest, back, stomach, legs, and feet. Using the hands as an example, begin by (a) tightening your hand muscles into fists. Notice the feeling of tension in your hands, wrists, and lower arms. Hold the tension for a few seconds, then (b) release your hands by relaxing your fists and letting the tension slip away. Notice how much lighter your hands feels than when tightened. Finally, (c) notice the difference between how your hands felt when tensed and how they felt when you released the tension. Enjoy the feeling of relaxation.
>
> **Stretching**. A simple way to loosen tight muscles and combat stress is to do

stretching exercises. They take only a few minutes and can be done at home or work. They will do you much more good than a coffee break. Some examples of stretching exercises are (a) **back stretch**—while sitting, stretch forward, rest your body on your lap, and relax your head and neck, letting your arms hang down. Hold for about a minute, then press on your thighs to help yourself sit up; (b) **neck stretch**—while standing or sitting, slowly tilt your head to the right without moving your shoulders, then slowly tilt it to the left; (c) **upper body stretch**—with your feet a comfortable distance apart, reach your hands overhead and stretch to the side (trying not to move your hips), then hold for 30 seconds and switch your hands to the other side; d) **leg stretch**—while standing, place one foot on a stool six or eight inches high and slowly lean forward, bending from your hips and keeping your back straight. For a full program, repeat each exercise five times.[27]

McBride points out that spiritual disciplines are important in treating stress.[28] For Christians the primary spiritual focus must be on the life and ministry of Jesus Christ, our role model. He faithfully carried out His mission despite tremendous trials and stresses. His life mission succeeded largely because of His devotional life. "Now in the morning, having risen a long while before daylight, He went out and departed to a solitary place; and there He prayed."[29] Jesus, it is recorded by Luke, "went out to the mountain to pray, and continued all night in prayer to God."[30] Each highlight and crisis in His life was connected to prayer. Jesus prayed at His baptism,[31] before His first confrontation with the Pharisees,[32] before He chose His disciples,[33] before He questioned His disciples as to who they thought He was,[34] at the Transfiguration,[35] and upon the cross.[36] Jesus, the divine Son of God, knew He could not live without prayer.

Another stress minimizer is peace—peace that exists despite toil and conflict. Christ makes these promises:

Peace I leave with you, My peace I give to you.[37]

The Lord will give strength to His people; the Lord will bless His people with peace.[38]

You will keep him in perfect peace, whose mind is stayed on You, because he trusts in You.[39]

These things I have spoken to you, that in Me you may have peace. In the world you will have tribulation; but be of good cheer, I have overcome the world.[40]

And the peace of God, which surpasses all understanding, will guard your hearts and minds through Christ Jesus.[41]

Sabbath keeping is a particularly good peace promoter. Another important aspect of peace is contentment. During his second imprisonment in Rome, the Apostle Paul wrote, "I have learned, in whatever state I am, to be content."[42] To the Corinthians, he wrote, "For the sake of Christ, then, I am content with weaknesses, insults, hardships, persecutions, and calamities; for when I am weak, then I am strong."[43]

Spiritual surrender also brings peace. Jesus experienced this in the Garden of Gethsemane as He prepared for the cross. His prayer was "not My will, but Yours be done."[44] As William Barclay writes,

> Life's hardest task is to accept what we cannot understand; but we can do even that if we are surrendered to God and are sure of His love.[45]

Positive Emotions

In a paper on stress control, Mark Finley emphasizes that we must develop positive emotions.[46] He suggests that gratitude, rejoicing, benevolence, and trust (faith) are health's greatest safeguards. An attitude of **thankfulness** goes a long way in reducing stress. We need to remain thankful even when misfortune comes."In everything give thanks; for this is the will of God in Christ Jesus for you."[47]

Rejoicing naturally associates with gratitude. This is not a superficial giddiness, but a deep, abiding happiness. Several years ago Blake Clark interviewed some of America's centenarians and found a common denominator. He said,

> Perhaps the key characteristic shared by most centenarians is a cheerful disposition, a feeling that things will work out for the best . . . songs and laughter somehow lubricate the biological clock and keep it running longer.[48]

Solomon said it well: "A merry heart does good like medicine, but a broken spirit dries the bones."[49]

A third positive emotion is **benevolence**—kindness and unselfishness. If each of us were a little more thoughtful and courteous each day, how much easier it would be to live in this stressful age. Selfishness destroys health; unselfishness promotes and imparts health.

Trust (faith) in a divine power "is a vitalizing attribute of the human mind which possesses tremendous psychic possibilities and extraordinary therapeutic powers. Tolstoy once called it 'the force of life'. . . . Faith calls for a complete and unconditional surrender of one's whole body, mind, and spirit to the idea which is believed in. Of necessity, it must further include obedience to that which it accepts."[50]

Positive emotions stimulate the parasympathetic nervous system, which largely controls digestion, absorption, elimination, circulation, and respiration; its activities dominate the support and recuperative functions of the body.[51] Stanford professor William Fry, Jr., is quoted saying that a good laugh (parasympathetic nervous system stimulation) can "aid digestion, lower blood pressure, stimulate the heart and endocrine system, activate the right brain hemisphere (your creative center), strengthen muscles, raise pulse rate, soothe arthritic pain, work out internal organs and keep you alert."[52] Richard Neil says that the average child laughs about 400 times per day; the average adult about 15 times. Jesus admonishes us to "become as little children."[53]

Paul summarized positive thinking in these terms:

Finally, brethren, whatever things are true, whatever things are noble, whatever things are just, whatever things are pure, whatever things are lovely, whatever things are of good report, if there is any virtue and if there is anything praiseworthy—meditate on these things.[54]

To the Romans, he urged,

Be kindly affectionate to one another with brotherly love, in honor giving preference to one another . . . rejoicing in hope, patient in tribulation . . . bless those who persecute you; bless and do not curse. Rejoice with those who rejoice, and weep with those who weep. . . . Repay no one evil for evil. Have regard for good things in the sight of all men. If it is possible, as much as depends on you, live peaceably with all men. Beloved, do not avenge yourselves.[55]

We *can* do all these things through Christ who strengthens us.[56]

Social Support

Isolation and its accompanying emotional pain are significant factors in much ill health. Dr. Dean Ornish has spoken eloquently of this problem. Ornish is best known for his lifestyle change program that has helped 82 percent of his patients with severe heart disease to reverse their coronary artery blockages. Recently he said,

I've been struck by the profound sense of isolation that so many people experience in our culture today—isolation from one's feelings, from other people, from the experience of something spiritual. By "spiritual," I mean the experience of feeling that while on one level we're separate, on another level we're all connected to each other and a part of something larger than ourselves.[57]

Ornish says studies around the world show that people who feel isolated have two to five times the incidence of disease and premature death as those who feel a sense of community with one another. In a recent prospective study, Dr. Lisa Berkman of Yale School of Medicine studied men and women who had recently suffered heart attacks. She simply asked them, "Can you count on anyone to provide you with emotional support?" The results were dramatic. People who answered "no" were almost three times as likely to die during the next six months as those who had at least one person providing emotional support.[58]

Ornish asks,

Why is social support so important? If you have no place that feels safe enough to let down your emotional walls and your defenses, then your barriers tend to remain up all the time. Unfortunately, the same walls that protect you can also isolate you if they are always up. . . . In our research, our support groups began as a place for people to exchange recipes, shopping tips, and so on, but it evolved into something much more powerful; a community, a place that felt safe enough for people to talk about what was really going on in their lives, what they were truly feeling, without fear of being judged, rejected, or abandoned.

Coping with the intensity of their pain is difficult for many people; frequently they turn to addictions or compulsive behavior as ways to drown loneliness.[59] Some of Ornish's patients have made statements like these:

- When something's eating me, I eat. When I'm lonely, which is most of the time, I eat. And then I eat some more. I keep trying to fill up the void with food.

- I smoke when I'm lonely. I've got twenty friends here in this pack of cigarettes, and they're always there for me. Nobody else is.

- I don't smoke, but I've got friends I see at the bar every day—Johnny Walker, Jim Beam, Old Grand Dad. They're always waiting for me. I drink to kill the pain.

- I keep busy. I never have enough time in the day. I'm always working. It distracts me from how lonely and unhappy I am. I feel such a letdown when I finish a project because it never brings me what I want most. Vacations are even harder because then I have the time to experience how lonely I feel.

- I channel-surf in front of the TV, switching from one channel to another to distract myself from my loneliness and emotional pain.

- My particular addiction, Ornish says, is talking on the telephone. For me, long distance is not only the next best thing to being there—sometimes it's even better. I can fill up the void and the loneliness without letting most people get *too* close.[60]

We become addicted to things that deaden our pain. Temporary pleasure hides the chronic pain, but it also tends to diminish the capacity to feel pleasure, joy, and love—for ourselves or others. Isolation may cause one to eat too much as a way of filling up the emotional emptiness and spiritual void. Eating may be used to address deeper spiritual needs.[61]

God sees our need for social and spiritual support and urges us "to consider one another in order to stir up love and good works, not forsaking the assembling of ourselves together, as is the manner of some, but exhorting one another, and so much the more as you see the Day approaching."[62]

Ornish points out that "many people don't find a feeling of community or meaning at church or synagogue, where the emphasis is often on the rituals rather than on the underlying spiritual meaning." How much more meaningful church could be if people felt free to express their problems, knowing they would receive genuine support from others. James urges, "Confess your trespasses to one another, and pray for one another, that you may be healed."[63] May God's church in these last days truly support those who suffer from emotional pain and the stresses of life. Our religion should be one of hope and comfort. "The eternal God is your refuge, and underneath are the everlasting arms. He will drive out your enemy from before you."[64] "Now may the God of hope fill you with all joy and peace in believing, that you may abound in hope by the power of the Holy Spirit."[65]

Mental Efficiency

Much of our discussion has centered on the thinking portion of the mind, the central nervous system, which is headed by the cerebral cortex. Weighing about three pounds, our complex brains are made up of more than 30 billion neurons (nerve cells) and five to ten times that number of glial support cells. The amount of information flooding into the brain through the eyes, ears, nose, and skin is staggering. The brain can cope only by selecting, by experience, what is important. If something dangerous happens, the brain instantly becomes alert. When a person slips on ice, for instance, the brain immediately signals how to regain balance or protect oneself in a fall. The event is stored in memory as a warning for more caution the next time.

Each nerve cell typically has a gray cell body topped by a sort of tree with numerous delicate branches (dendrites), through which the neuron receives signals from other cells. On each neuron is a long, white-sheathed tail called an axon, which transmits nerve impulses to terminals. A single axon may branch into as many as 10,000 terminals, each of which can connect to separate neurons. Since each neuron can receive signals from more than a thousand other neurons, a single nerve cell could conceivably carry on several million separate conversations at the same time. It's a mind-boggling feat, especially considering the astronomical number of neurons in the brain.

Neurons never actually touch one another. When a nerve impulse reaches an axon terminal, it releases a packet of message-bearing chemicals (neurotransmitters). These jump a tiny gap (synapse) and fit into the protein receptors on the dendrites of the receiving cells. The neurotransmitters can either be excitatory or inhibitory; stimulating the receiving cell to produce an electrical impulse or preventing it from firing. If a cell receives sufficient excitation in enough dendrites, it fires, and the electrical impulse flashes down the axon to release specific neuro-transmitters at its tip. Then the process potentially continues across another synapse.[66] These nerve impulses travel along nerve cells at speeds up to 225 miles per hour.[67]

Neurons constantly make new connections or rearrange old circuits in our brains. New experiences appear to activate specific parts of the brain which develop enriched networks of brain cells. Everything a person ever does or expe-riences leaves its mark in the brain cells, influencing their growth and connections. Both your genetic endowment and the effects of your culture are engraved in every cell. Each individual, therefore, sees a unique picture of the world.[68]

Physiologically, "thought probably results from the momentary 'pattern' of stimulation of many different parts of the nervous system all at the same time, probably involving most importantly the cerebral cortex, the thalamus, the limbic system, and the upper reticular formation of the brain stem. . . . Consciousness can perhaps be described as our continuing stream of awareness of either our surroundings or our sequential thoughts. . . . Memory must be equally as complex as the mechanism of a thought, for, to provide memory, the nervous system must recreate the same pattern" as in the original thought.[69]

The complexity of the central nervous system helps us realize the turmoil of the unguided mind and understand how the devil allows his followers "no rest day or night." The greatest blessing of following God is the reassurance that He guides our minds.

I will instruct and teach you in the way you should go; I will guide you with My eye.[70]

For God has not given us a spirit of fear, but of power and of love and of a sound *mind*.[71]

If any of you lacks wisdom, let him ask of God, who gives to all liberally and without reproach, and it will be given to him.[72]

It is God who works in you both to will and to do for His good pleasure.[73]

And the peace of God, which surpasses all understanding, will guard your hearts and *minds* through Christ Jesus.[74]

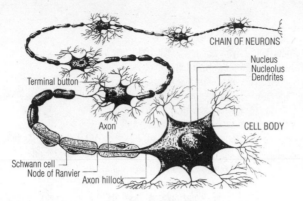

Figure 6. *A nerve pathway showing six neurons and the axons connecting with the dendrites of the next cell.*

Uncertainty about decisions causes stress as the mind seeks to develop new pathways of thought. Wondering whether you "should do this or that" causes the nerve paths to go round and round. The mind cannot rest until satisfactory pathways are established. Good habits result from settled pathways which are not associated with any ill effects. Bad habits also result from well-developed paths, but they may disturb the conscience or lead to harmful actions. Clearly, good habits are a more efficient use of the brain. God's design for a clear mind is that we keep His law on our hearts.

> The law of the Lord is perfect, converting the soul; the testimony of the Lord is sure, making wise the simple; the statutes of the Lord are right, rejoicing the heart; the commandment of the Lord is pure, enlightening the eyes; the fear of the Lord is clean, enduring forever; the judgments of the Lord are true and righteous altogether.[75]

> Your word is a lamp to my feet and a light to my path.[76]

> I delight to do Your will, O my God, and Your law is within my heart.[77]

Prayer of Consecration

God, let me rest fully in You and enjoy the pleasant thoughts with which You fill my mind. You have promised, "Do not fear, little flock, for it is your Father's good pleasure to give you the kingdom."[78] Thank you, Lord. I've had enough of the world's restlessness. Reign in my heart, for that is my desire. Amen.

1 Revelation 14:11.
2 "Don't Let Stress Number Your Days," *Longevity* Oct. 1990: 50.
3 John Marks, "Time Out," *U. S. News & World Report* 11 Dec. 1995: 85-97.
4 Flora Johnson Skelly, "Stress Busters," *American Medical News* 24/31 Oct. 1994: 15.
5 "A Guide to Managing Stress," *Health Information Library* (Krames Communications) 2.
6 Carol A. and Louis R. Torres, *Notes on Music* (Creation Enterprises International, 1991) and
   Lowell Hart, *Satan's Music Exposed* (Salem Kirban Inc., 1981).
7 Gervasia M. Schrockenberg and Harvey H. Bird, "Neural Plasticity of MUS musculus in Response to
   Disharmonic Sound," *Bulletin of the New Jersey Academy of Science,* vol. 32, no. 2, Fall 1987.
8 J. Michael McGinnis, "Behavior Patterns and Health," *Medicine for the Layman* (NIH Publication No. 85-
   2682, 1985) 33.
9 Lydia Woods Schindler, *The Immune System: How it Works* (NIH Publication No. 92-3229, June 1992).
10 J. Michael McGinnis, "Behavior Patterns and Health," *Medicine for the Layman* (NIH Publication No. 85-
   2682, 1985).
11 Tracy B. Herbert, "Stress and the Immune System," *World Health* Mar.-April 1994: 4, 5.
12 Dr. Ali Husein, "Exploring the Mind and Spirit," *World Health* Mar.-April 1994: 8.
13 Carey and Bruno, "Why Cynicism Can Be Fatal," *Newsweek* 10 Sept. 1984: 68.
14 Doneta Wrate, "Stress: How Does Your Way of Coping Affect Your Physical Health," *Natural Lifestyle and
   Your Health* Oct. 1994.
15 David C. Nieman, DHSc, "The Mind and Health," *The Adventist Healthstyle* (Review & Herald Publishing,
   1992) 104.
16 Gurney Williams III, "Hopping-Heart-Stopping-Mad: Why Blowing Up May Up Your Risk of a Heart Attack,"
   Longevity Aug. 1944: 28.
17 Ephesians 4:26, 27, 29, 31, 32.
18 Edward Dolnick, "Hotheads and Heart Attacks," *Health* July/Aug. 1995: 58-64.
19 Peter McWilliams, "Happiness . . . Understanding Happiness," *Bottom Line Personal* 15 Jan. 1993: 1, 2.
20 Proverbs 23:7.
21 Hans Selye, *The Stress of Life* (McGraw Hill Book Co., 1956) 284.
22 Ellen G. White, *Ministry of Healing* (Pacific Press, 1909) 251.
23 Ibid, 241.
24 John W. Farquhar, MD, "Stress and How to Cope With It," *The American Way of Life Need Not Be Hazardous
   to Your Health"* (W. W. Norton & Co., 1978) 57-79.
25 Flora Johnson Skelly, "Stress Busters," *American Medical News* 24/31 Oct. 1994: 16.
26 Raymond B. Flannery Jr, PhD, "Towards Stress-Resistant Persons: A Stress Management Approach to the
   Treatment of Anxiety," *American Journal of Preventive Medicine,* vol. 3, no. 1, 1987: 25-30.
27 Kate C. Ross, "A Guide to Managing Stress," *Health Information Library* (Krames Communications, 1985).
28 Michael G. McBride, "Managing Ministerial Stress," *Ministry* Mar. 1989: 8-11.
29 Mark 1:35.
30 Luke 6:12.
31 Luke 3:21.
32 Luke 5:16.
33 Luke 6:12, 13.
34 Luke 9:18.
35 Luke 9:29.
36 Luke 23:34.
37 John 14:27.

[38] Psalm 29:11.

[39] Isaiah 26:3.

[40] John 16:33.

[41] Philippians 4:7.

[42] Philippians 4:11.

[43] 2 Corinthians 12:10 (RSV).

[44] Luke 22:42.

[45] William Barclay, *The Gospel of Mark* (Westminster Press, 1956).

[46] Mark Finley, "Strategy for Stress Control," undated, unpublished paper.

[47] 1 Thessalonians 5:18.

[48] Blake Clark, *Reader's Digest* Feb. 1976: 132.

[49] Proverbs 17:22.

[50] William S. Sadler, MD, "Philosophy of Life," *Mental Mischief and Emotional Conflict* (C.V. Mosby Co., 1947) 371.

[51] Mervyn G. Hardinge, "Emotions," *A Philosophy of Health* (LLU School of Health syllabus, 1980) 154.

[52] William F. Frye, "Why Laughing is Good for Your Health," *Healing Unlimited* (Boardroom Classics, 1995) 411.

[53] Richard L. Neil, MD, "Stress Through the Ages," a lecture given on March 2, 1990, at the Update Convention of the School of Public Health of Loma Linda University.

[54] Philippians 4:8.

[55] Romans 12:10, 12-15, 17-19.

[56] Philippians 4:13.

[57] Dean Ornish, "Isolation . . . and Your Heart," *Bottom Line Personal* 15 July 1992: 11.

[58] Dean Ornish, "What's Eating You?" *Eat More, Weigh Less* (Harper Perrenial, 1993) 62.

[59] Ibid, 63, 64.

[60] Ibid, 65, 66.

[61] Ibid, 66-70.

[62] Hebrews 10:24, 25.

[63] James 5:16.

[64] Deuteronomy 33:27 (KJV).

[65] Romans 15:13.

[66] "Landscapes of the Mind," *The Incredible Machine* (National Geographic Society, 1986) 325-375.

[67] J. D. Ratcliff, "Central Nervous System," *I Am Joe's Body* (A Berkley/Reader's Digest Book, 1980) 11-16.

[68] Ibid, 345.

[69] Arthur C. Guyton, MD, "Cerebral Cortex and Intellectual Functions of the Brain," *Human Physiology and Mechanisms of Disease,* 4th ed. (W. B. Saunders Co, 1987) 415-423.

[70] Psalm 32:8.

[71] 2 Timothy 1:7.

[72] James 1:5.

[73] Philippians 2:13.

[74] Philippians 4:7.

[75] Psalm 19:7-9.

[76] Psalm 119:105.

[77] Psalm 40:8.

[78] Luke 12:32.

Chapter Eleven

Patience
of the Saints

Here is the patience of the saints; here are those who keep the command-ments of God. Revelation 14:12.

The third angel ends his fearful message with a beautiful description of the worshipers of God. The verse begins, "Here is the patience of the saints; here are they that keep the commandments of God. . . ."[1] Knowing the dreadful end of the wicked, God's people feel a renewed, stronger desire to serve Him. The paraphrase of the Living Bible says, "Let this encourage God's people to endure patiently every trial and persecution, for they are His saints who remain firm to the end in obedience to His commands. . . ." The Clear Word paraphrase says, "These things that I saw will call for special endurance on the part of God's people who keep the commandments of God. . . ."

Patience refers to steadfast endurance—a type of discipline—and specifically includes keeping the "commandments of God." This is a good description of the process of sanctification, the goal of all Christians. "As you therefore have received Christ Jesus the Lord, so walk in Him, rooted and built up in Him and established in the faith. . . ."[2] The high goal is to "stand perfect and complete in all the will of God."[3] Jesus Himself set the standard: "Therefore you shall be perfect, just as your Father in heaven is perfect."[4] To be "perfect and complete" clearly includes the whole person—body, mind, and soul.

The Spiritual Value of Self-restraint

Sanctification involves the proper care of our bodies. Paul writes,

For this is the will of God, your sanctification: that you should abstain from sexual immorality; that each of you should know how to possess his own vessel [body] in sanctification and honor, not in passion of lust, like the Gentiles who do not know God. . . . For God did not call us to uncleanness, but in holiness.[5]

"Works of the flesh," from which we are to abstain, are graphically listed by Paul:

> Now the works of the flesh are evident, which are: adultery, fornication, uncleanness, lewdness, idolatry, sorcery, hatred, contentions, jealousies, outbursts of wrath, selfish ambitions, dissensions, heresies, envy, murders, drunkenness, revelries, and the like; of which I tell you beforehand, just as I also told you in time past, that those who practice such things will not inherit the kingdom of God.[6]

Paul encourages the Romans, "For if you live according to the flesh you will die; but if by the Spirit you put to death the deeds of the body, you will live."[7]

God never tells us it will be easy. In fact, He calls this special discipline "suffering," and suggests we should "joy in" and "rejoice in" the suffering that builds character and prepares us for God's kingdom.

> My brethren, count it *all joy* when you fall into various trials, knowing that the testing of your faith produces patience. But let patience have its perfect work, that you may be perfect and complete, lacking nothing.[8]

> And not only that, but we also *glory in tribulations*, knowing that tribulation produces perseverance; and perseverance, character; and character, hope. Now hope does not disappoint, because the love of God has been poured out in our hearts by the Holy Spirit who was given to us.[9]

The discipline (suffering) of the present is nothing compared with the glory God plans to show through us.[10]

The value of this self-discipline (restraint) is recognized even by secular authors. In a book on weight control, it is pointed out that dietary restrictions exist in all cultures and religions.

> Some religions forbid pork; others allow it. Some religions dictate fasting on certain days and feasting on others. Yet even though the specific dietary guidelines vary in each religion, all of them are designed to bring us closer to God. Does God care or are these dietary restrictions for us?

> While there may be inherent benefit in each religion's recommendations, I believe that just the act of having voluntary restraints is beneficial to us. When we choose not to eat something when we might otherwise do so, the effect is to make the act of eating more special, more sacred, and thus more joyful. Also, voluntary restraint helps us to break free of our compulsions and our addictions.

> Why not just do everything you want? Why impose limitations on your freedom? Because *self-imposed* limitations can help to free us.

For example, if a musician spends several hours a day practicing, it may seem as though she is limiting her freedom. She could be doing so many other things. But this self-discipline gives her the power and freedom to express herself through her music in ways that many others cannot. We all understand the value of self-discipline for an athlete who spends hours a day training intensely for the Olympics. Yet we may find it more difficult to understand the spiritual value of self-restraint.

When we understand the benefits of our choices, then they become easier to make. What appears like self-restraint can be self-empowerment. Ultimately, it's a choice between true freedom or being a slave to our compulsions.[11]

Understanding its value makes it easier for us to rejoice in self-discipline.

Jesus, Our Example

We are told that He, the "captain of our salvation," was made "perfect through suffering."[12] He learned obedience—self-discipline—even as we must. "Though He was a Son [the Son of God], yet He learned obedience by the things which He suffered. And having been perfected, He became the author of eternal salvation to all who obey Him."[13]

Of the first 30 years of Jesus' life, we have little record. We know he lived in the wicked town of Nazareth.[14] He was obedient ("subject to") His parents.[15] He grew and developed a symmetrical, balanced life. "And Jesus increased in wisdom and stature, and in favor with God and men."[16] Because His parents were poor, Jesus worked in His father's shop and gained a reputation as a carpenter.[17] I can imagine the care with which He worked—smoothing the boards, making clean, tight joints and square corners, working with exactness and self-restraint.

There are few disciplines that teach self-control better than hard physical labor. Making every muscle work exactly as desired requires long practice and accurate use of the nervous system and muscles. It is rigorous discipline that carries over into many other parts of life.

At the creation, **labor** was appointed as a blessing. It meant development, power, happiness. . . . Though now attended with anxiety, weariness, and pain, it is still a source of happiness and development. And it is a safeguard against temptation. Its discipline places a check on self-indulgence, and promotes industry, purity, and firmness. Thus it [manual labor] becomes a part of God's great plan for our recovery from the Fall.[18]

Jesus also engaged in the discipline of study and memorization of **God's Word**. He resisted most of Satan's temptations with an "It is written" and an appropriate Scripture text that He had memorized. His other lesson book was **nature**. He illustrated deep things of God with parables which could easily be understood by

His listeners. Finally, as discussed in Chapter 9, Jesus lived in close relationship with His Father in Heaven through many hours of **prayer and meditation**. His discipline prepared Him to completely surrender His will to God. "Not My will, but Yours, be done."[19] "And being found in appearance as a man, He humbled himself and became obedient to the point of death, even the death of the cross."[20]

Jesus is our ultimate example of discipline, self-restraint, and obedience.

"Works" and Salvation

The third angel describes God's people as saints who patiently endure discipline. They are next described as being those who "keep the commandments of God." Are they saved by their works of commandment keeping? Decidedly not!

For by *grace* you have been saved through faith, and that not of yourselves; *it is the gift of God, not of works*, lest anyone should boast. For we are His workmanship, created in Christ Jesus for good works, which God prepared beforehand that we should walk in them.[21]

It couldn't be stated more clearly. We are saved "by grace" and "not of works," for "it is the gift of God." However, we are "created in Christ Jesus for good works." The "good works" include keeping the commandments of God.

Why do God's children keep the commandments? Most importantly, Christians love God for who He is and what He has done for us. Jesus said, "If you love Me, keep My commandments."[22] Secondly, because we were created for the "good works" of keeping the commandments—"to walk in them,"[23] no longer "as the rest of the Gentiles walk," but "renewed in the spirit of your mind . . . that you put on the new man which was created according to God, in true righteousness and holiness."[24]

"Righteousness and holiness" include keeping God's commandments, not because we are forced to, but because we love God. Lovers always seek to please the one they love. They also want to stay close to their loved one. Jesus said, "If you love Me, keep My commandments. And I will pray the Father, and He will give you another Helper (Comforter), that He may abide with you forever—the Spirit of truth, whom the world cannot receive, because it neither sees Him nor knows Him; but you know Him, for He dwells with you and will be in you."[25] There can be no closer relationship than God, our Lover, in us.

Why does God desire us to keep His commandments? First, because He desires for us the good things that come only as we obey His wise laws. "My son, do not forget my law, but let your heart keep my commands; for length of days and long life and peace they will add to you . . . fear the Lord and depart from evil. It will be health to your flesh, and strength to your bones."[26]

Secondly, God chooses to show His glory through us. In the theater of the universe, we are His actors. "The creation eagerly waits for the revealing of the sons of God."[27]

For our best good, God has given us at least three sets of laws. They demonstrate His love and how we can reveal Him most clearly to others.

- The Ten Commandment **moral law** is over all, clarifying our relationship both to God and man.

- Related to the Ten Commandments is God's **natural law,** which governs the actions of our human bodies. By keeping these laws, we also keep the moral law, which declares, "You shall not murder [kill]."[28] By purposely harming my body, I am guilty of killing. In respect for my Creator, I will care for His creation.

- As an expansion of the moral law, God gave the children of Israel **social (civil) laws** to assist in their governance. These civil laws remain the foundation for current law in most nations.

God's perfect law of liberty encompasses these three. Of it, James writes:

But he who looks into the perfect law of liberty and continues in it, and is not a forgetful hearer but a doer of the work, this one will be blessed in what he does.[29]

Preparation for Heaven

God is preparing people today to go with Him to heaven. Consider the parallel between what God does for us today and what He did to help the children of Israel on their way to the Promised Land. "Now all these things happened to them as examples, and they were written for our admonition, upon whom the ends of the ages have come."[30]

The first promise given to the children of Israel after they crossed the Red Sea on their way to Canaan was this:

If you diligently heed the voice of the Lord your God and do what is right in His sight, give ear to His commandments and keep all His statutes, I will put none of the diseases on you which I have brought on the Egyptians. For I am the Lord who heals you.[31]

This first message was a health message, and it was so important that it was repeated later in Exodus: "I will take sickness away from the midst of you."

The first message God gave the Seventh-day Adventist Church after its organization in May, 1863, was a health message.[32] It clarified that God wishes to be glorified by the life and health of His people. Health, however, is dependent on following the laws God has written in our bodies—the laws of health. Health messages were often given to Ellen White, and sometimes they were repeated to emphasize their significance.

Dietary reform, health rules, and laws of sanitation and hygiene were specifically given to the children of Israel as a part of their preparation for the Promised Land. God has blessed His people in these last days with a comprehensive health message, beautifully encapsulated in the book *Ministry of Healing*. God makes it clear that He is not satisfied with soul prosperity alone:

> Beloved, I pray that you may prosper in all things and be in health, just as your soul prospers.[33]

God desired that the children of Israel be set "high above all nations of the earth. . . . The Lord will establish you as a holy people to Himself. . . . Then all peoples of the earth shall see that you are called by the name of the Lord. . . . And the Lord will make you the head and not the tail."[34] In these last days we are told that "the creation eagerly waits for the revealing of the sons of God," who are designated to be "a spectacle to the world."[35]

Finally, God is merciful even to those who don't deserve it. He promised to protect the health of the children of Israel. Despite their waywardness and disobedience, "He brought them out with silver and gold, and there was none feeble among His tribes." Why did God give them health? "That they might observe His statutes and keep His laws. Praise the Lord!"[36]

Adventist Health Studies

Scientific studies of Seventh-day Adventists around the world have shown they have less illness, lower mortality, and greater longevity than the general population. This is true despite the failure of many Seventh-day Adventists to live healthy lifestyles. God remains merciful to His people.

The first report on the health of Adventists to appear in peer-reviewed scientific literature was published in 1958. It showed that Adventists in California appeared to have considerably less cancer and heart disease than the general population. This stimulated great interest in the Adventist lifestyle. More than $10 million in research grants from the National Institutes of Health alone has gone into studies of Adventists in California. Studies have also been done on the health of Adventists from Australia, New Zealand, Japan, the Netherlands, Norway, Poland, and the Caribbean islands, as well as the U.S. More than 250 reports on Adventists have appeared in the scientific literature of the world. No other religious group has attracted more interest from scientists.

The 1958 Adventist study in California involved 25,000 church members, who have been followed for more than 30 years. In 1974 another 35,000 Adventist households in California were enrolled in an ongoing study. The results of this research have profoundly affected health recommendations given around the world. Here are some of the most important findings from the California Adventist Study:

- The average life expectancy of a 35-year-old Adventist male is 47.0 additional years of life (8.9 years longer than the average California male); the corresponding difference for a 35-year-old Adventist female is 7.5 years.[37]

- 20 percent of Adventists in California eat meat more than four times a week; 55 percent are lacto-ovo vegetarians. When Adventists who eat meat are compared with those who do not, the following is found: Adventist males 45 to 64 years old who eat meat have a threefold greater risk of fatal heart attack than those who do not eat meat;[38] 40-year-old Adventist male vegetarians outlive non-vegetarians by 3.7 years.[39]

- Death rates for all cancer for Adventists are 56 percent of what is expected at California rates (for same age and sex); for lung cancer, Adventists have 25 percent the expected rate; for colon cancer, 49 percent. Adventist women have 83 percent the expected rate of breast cancer.[40]

- For coronary occlusions (fatal heart attacks), Adventists have 43 percent (less than half) as many as expected at California rates; for cerebral strokes, it is 48 percent.

- For deaths from all causes, Adventists have 49 percent the death rate expected in California. (This means that only half as many Adventists die each year as expected, which reconciles with the fact that Adventists live significantly longer. Adventists eventually die of diseases similar to the rest of Californians; they just die at an older age.)

- In a recently published long-term study comparing 4,342 Loma Linda University (LLU) medical school graduates with 2,832 medical school graduates from the University of Southern California (USC), the death rates for LLU physicians were 42 percent lower than among USC physicians. The groups were similar socioeconomically, and neither group smoked significantly. The principal differences were that the USC physicians consumed more meat, eggs, coffee, and alcohol and fewer fruits and legumes than did the LLU physicians.[41]

Despite the fact that many Seventh-day Adventists have not lived up to the health message given to the church, God has been merciful, and church members enjoy better health than the general population. This has been proved true in every country where Adventist health studies have been conducted. What could God reveal through us if we took seriously the responsibility to glorify God in our bodies?

While the avoidance of alcohol and tobacco is responsible for most health advantages seen in Adventists, it is clear that diet, exercise, and other factors improve survival. Nieman points out that

> the Adventist lifestyle boils down to trust in God, daily moderate outdoor exercise, regular and sufficient rest, avoidance of harmful substances, and a healthy lacto-ovovegetarian diet. It is curious that so many SDAs (Seventh-day Adventists) have not made the decision to fully enter into this lifestyle.[42]

Evidence shows that Adventists are tending to move away from a vegetarian diet just as many in the general population are adopting this more healthful lifestyle.

God has graciously given us bodies, and we may do with them as we desire. It is His plan for us to use these bodies to practice the lifestyle of heaven. May our love for Him motivate us to keep His laws of health. May His glory be revealed to the world through us.

Prayer

Your way of life is good, Lord. The discipline you would have us follow leads to improved health and strength. Thank you for Your mercy in blessing our feeble efforts to live your lifestyle. Make us shining examples and use us to draw others to You. Glorify us so we can glorify You. Amen.

---

[1] Revelation 14:12.
[2] Colossians 2:6, 7.
[3] Colossians 4:12, last part.
[4] Matthew 5:48.
[5] 1 Thessalonians 4:3-5, 7.
[6] Galatians 5:19-21.
[7] Romans 8:13.
[8] James 1:2-4.
[9] Romans 5:3-5.
[10] Romans 8:18, 19.
[11] Dean Ornish, MD, "Who You Are Is Not What You Weigh," *Eat More, Weigh Less* (Harper Perrenial, 1993) 73, 74.
[12] Hebrews 2:10.
[13] Hebrews 5:8, 9.
[14] John 1:46.
[15] Luke 2:51.
[16] Luke 2:52.
[17] Mark 6:3.
[18] Ellen G. White, *Education* (Pacific Press, 1903) 214.
[19] Luke 22:42.
[20] Philippians 2:8.
[21] Ephesians 2:8-10.
[22] John 14:15.

23 Ephesians 2:10.
24 Ephesians 4:17, 23, 24.
25 John 14:15-17.
26 Psalm 3:1, 2, 7, 8.
27 Romans 8:19.
28 Exodus 20:13; Deuteronomy 5:17.
29 James 1:25.
30 1 Corinthians 10:11.
31 Exodus 15:26.
32 Note: The first and largest health vision given Ellen G. White was given less than two weeks after the General Conference which first established the organization of the Seventh-day Adventist church.
33 3 John 2.
34 Deuteronomy 28:1, 9, 10, 13.
35 Romans 8:19; 1 Corinthians 4:9.
36 Psalm 105:37, 45.
37 Jan W. Kuzma, "Adventists and Good Health," *Adventist Review* 29 June 1989: 17.
38 David C. Nieman, DHSc, "The Adventist Health Study," *The Adventist Healthstyle* (Review & Herald, 1992) 36, 39.
39 Kuzma, Ibid, 18.
40 Strahan, Stanton, and Fraser, "Adventist Health Studies," *AIMS Study Guide* (Creation Enterprises International, 1991) 8-11. (This citation is for all disease-specific death rates listed.)
41 *Journal of the American Medical Association* 265 (1991) 2352-2359.
42 David C. Nieman, Ibid, 41.

CHAPTER TWELVE

The Faith of Jesus

HERE ARE THOSE WHO KEEP . . . THE FAITH OF JESUS. REVELATION 14:12 (LAST PART).

T he third angel's call to worship ends with a glorious description of true worshipers. As described in the last chapter, they are those who are stead- fast, patiently enduring the discipline necessary to make disciples. They keep God's commandments and live pure lives that show the universe what God is like. But they don't do this alone; it is by their faith in Jesus.

The King James, New King James, and Revised Standard versions of the Bible speak of keeping "the faith *of* Jesus." Most other translations speak of "faith *in* Jesus." The faith *of* Jesus is the faith He had in His Father, which is the same faith we must have *in* Jesus. Jesus said, "No one comes to the Father except through Me. If you had known Me, you would have known My father also."[1] He further promises, "If anyone loves Me, he will keep My word; and My Father will love him, and We will come to him and make Our home with him."[2] Our only hope of heaven is "Christ [through His Spirit] in you, the hope of glory . . . that we may present every man perfect in Christ Jesus."[3] Our perfection can only be by Christ *in* us and we *in* Christ.

Righteousness By Faith

Theologians and Christian philosophers have all wrestled with the great ques- tion, "What must I do to be saved?" The debate centers mainly on whether we are saved by faith in Christ or by our works. The non-Christian world almost univer- sally lives by works; they earn merit or otherwise satisfy their gods by good deeds. Christian legalists also view salvation as if it were earned by keeping God's commandments. Study of God's law—His natural law in our bodies—teaches the importance of balance between faith and works. It is not reasonable to ask God to heal if we are not being responsible in obeying His natural laws. On the other hand, we need faith in God and His power to enable us to obey. The Bible and human experience make this quite clear.

Jesus told Paul on the Damascus road, you "are sanctified by faith in Me."[4] He told the Galatians that "the life I now live in the flesh I live by faith in the Son of

God."[5] Our righteousness is not "from the law, but that which is through faith in Christ."[6] "Whoever calls on the name of the Lord shall be saved."[7] By believing "that Jesus is the Christ, the Son of God . . . you may have life in His name." Peter exclaimed, "There is no other name under heaven given among men by which we must be saved."[8]

In the context of eating, Paul says that "whatever is not from faith is sin."[9] What, then, is our work when faith in Christ is so strongly pointed to as our salvation? Paul reminds us that faith *is* work. He remembers the Thessalonians' "work of faith."[10] The question was asked, "What shall we do, that we may work the works of God?" and Jesus answered, "This is the work of God, that you believe in Him whom He sent."[11] Our "work" is to yield ourselves, including our bodies, fully to Christ, "believing in Him."

This includes some "doing," in His strength. "This is His commandment: that we should believe on the name of His Son Jesus Christ and love one another."[12] James reminds us, "Faith, by itself, if it does not have works, is dead. But someone will say, 'You have faith, and I have works.' Show me your faith without your works, and I will show you my faith by my works." And James adds that "by works faith was made perfect."[13]

Again, I say, our *work* is the discipline to constantly, minute-by-minute, place our will in God's hands, having the faith to believe that God will finish the work. The promises that He will do this are abundant.

Work out your own salvation with fear and trembling; for *it is God who works in you both to will and to do* His good pleasure.[14]

Trust in the Lord, and do good. . . . *He shall bring forth your righteousness.*[15]

Now may the God of peace *Himself sanctify you completely*; and may your whole spirit, soul, and body be preserved blameless at the coming of our Lord Jesus Christ. He who calls you is faithful, *who also will do it*.[16]

We also eagerly wait for the Savior, the Lord Jesus Christ, *who will transform* our lowly body that it may be conformed to His glorious body, according to the working by which *He is able* even to subdue all things to Himself.[17]

[We] shall be like Him, for we shall see Him as He is. And everyone who has this hope in Him purifies himself, just as He is pure.[18]

I can do all things through *Christ who strengthens me*.[19]

Now to *Him who is able* to do exceedingly abundantly above all that we ask or think, according to the power that works in us, to Him be glory in the church by Christ Jesus to all generations, forever and ever. Amen.[20]

Motivation for Health

The body broken down into its chemical constituents has little monetary value. Why does God speak so much about health in the Bible? Why does He urge us to give our bodies to Him,[21] speak of them as holy and to be cared for under penalty of death,[22] and urge us to glorify Him in our bodies?[23] Why should we take special interest in our bodies?

Most people seek health for poor motives. They wish to avoid discomfort or pain, they are afraid of death, or they simply want more years of life. Perhaps their desire for power over others is so strong that they try to maintain health in order to retain power. Others may be motivated by desire for beauty and strong muscles. In teaching health we must begin with whatever motives people have, but we need to encourage higher and stronger motives.

The highest motives for good health relate to our relationship with God. Powerful incentives are provided by these motives:

- I want to assist God in His effort to restore His image in me.

- I want a healthy body to support a strong, clear mind able to discern between truth and error.

- I desire a clean, well-maintained body temple for God's Spirit to dwell in.

- I recognize that worshiping God includes serving others, especially the most needy. To succeed in this work requires a strong and courageous body and mind.

- I want to show the world that God's natural laws are rational and reasonable. I want to demonstrate this picture of God in the way I treat my body.

- God has been so good to me that I love Him and desire to do whatever He wants.

- I desire to show the world God's way in contrast with Satan's. Then all may clearly differentiate and be able to make their final choices for God or Satan.

NEWSTART

The beauty of God's plan is its balance and simplicity. It does not require expensive resources; in fact, even the poorest can enjoy God's recommended lifestyle. If we cooperate with Him, God can bless His natural methods and restore health. We must remember, though, that health is not earned; it is God's gift to those who seek to follow His plan.

Together with David we can praise God, who is just as willing to heal our diseases as to forgive our sins.

> Bless the Lord, O my soul, and forget not all His benefits: who forgives all your iniquities, who heals all your diseases, who redeems your life from destruction, who crowns you with loving-kindness and tender mercies, who satisfies your mouth with good things, so that your youth is renewed like the eagle's. . . . As a father pities his children, so the Lord pities those who fear Him. For He knows our frame; He remembers that we are dust. As for man, his days are like grass; as a flower of the field, so he flourishes, for the wind passes over it and it is gone. And its place remembers it no more. But the mercy of the Lord is from everlasting to everlasting on those who fear Him, and His righteousness to children's children, to such as keep His covenant, and to those who remember His commandments to do them.[24]

God is able to heal, but considers it only reasonable that we cooperate by "remembering His commandments to do them," not to earn health, but because of our loving desire to follow Him. Weimar Institute's NEWSTART acronym provides a good reminder of God's ways:

Nutrition

Exercise

Water

Sunshine

Temperance

Air

Rest

Trust in God

While God expects us to use His simple, natural remedies, we need to understand that it is not a denial of faith to use medicine or surgery in case of serious illness. God can work through many remedial agencies. He could have healed Hezekiah by His word, but he chose to work through a fig poultice to bring about the king's healing.[25] We need to stay close enough (and quiet enough) to hear His voice when "your ears shall hear a word behind you, saying, 'This is the way, walk in it,' whenever you turn to the right hand or whenever you turn to the left."[26]

The same James who admonished prayer for the sick (James 5) is the one who points out that "every good gift and every perfect gift is from above, and comes down from the Father of lights, from whom there is no variation or shadow of turning."[27] Whatever happens, remember it is allowed by God, the only one who knows the end from the beginning. We must keep in mind that "all things work together for good to those who love God, to those who are the called according to His purpose."[28]

Restoration

We are living in "the times of restoration of all things, which God has spoken of by the mouth of all His holy prophets since the world began."[29] God is seeking to restore in us His image. We should pray, "Restore to me the joy of Your salvation, and uphold me by Your generous Spirit. Then I will teach transgressors Your ways, and sinners shall be converted to You."[30] God seeks joy for us that others might see His way as desirable. He desires that "in all things God may be glorified through Christ Jesus, to whom belong the glory and the dominion forever and ever. Amen."[31]

The third angel calls us to have faith in the God of the superlatives. Speaking of His sheep (us), Jesus said, "I have come that they may have life." Life is a wonderful gift, but Jesus didn't come that we might have ordinary life. He added, "I have come that they might have life *more abundantly*."[32] Paul seemed to be carried away with this God of superlatives, as he prayed "that He would grant you, according to the riches of His glory, to be strengthened with might through His Spirit in the inner man, that Christ may dwell in your heart through faith . . . that you may be able . . . to know the love of Christ which passes knowledge, that you may be filled with all the fullness of God." And then Paul really gets into the superlatives. "Now to Him who is *able to do exceedingly abundantly above all that we ask or think,* according to the power that works in us, to Him be gory in the church by Christ Jesus to all generations forever and ever. Amen."[33]

I believe the most profound testimony to what God will do through His children on earth is written by Ellen G. White in *Ministry of Healing.* She, like Paul, is overcome by the immensity of what God is waiting to do through us. She writes:

> The humblest workers, in cooperation with Christ, may touch chords whose vibrations shall ring to the ends of the earth, and make melody throughout eternal ages.

> Heavenly intelligences are waiting to cooperate with human instrumentalities, that they may reveal to the world what human beings may become, and what, through union with the Divine, may be accomplished for the saving of souls that are ready to perish. There is no limit to the usefulness of one who, putting self aside, makes room for the working of the Holy Spirit upon his heart, and lives a life wholly consecrated to God. All who consecrate body, soul, and spirit to His service will be constantly receiving a new endowment of physical, mental, and spiritual power. The inexhaustible supplies of heaven are at their command. Christ gives them the breath of His own Spirit, the life of His own life. The Holy Spirit puts forth its highest energies to work in mind and heart. Through the grace

given us we may achieve victories that because of our own erroneous and preconceived opinions, our defects of character, our smallness of faith, have seemed impossible.

To every one who offers himself to the Lord for service, withholding nothing, is given power for the attainment of measureless results. For these God will do great things. He will work upon the minds of men so that, even in this world, there shall be seen in their lives a fulfillment of the promise of the future state.[34]

The Final Act in the Drama of the Ages

God seeks in the messages of Revelation 14 to tell "every nation, tribe, tongue, and people" of the everlasting gospel and its application to the end time. Through the first angel, He makes Himself known. He tells who He is and how to "give glory to Him." It is a solemn time because "the hour of His judgment has come"—the time when each person makes a final decision for or against God.

The second angel has good news: "Babylon is fallen." The victory of Christ over Satan has been gained, but most of the world does not yet understand this. The original temptation for humans—to be their own gods—remains an overwhelming temptation for most people. Sexual impurity, intoxicating drinks, and harmful drugs allure many today.

The third angel tells of Satan's horrendous effort to convince the world to worship falsely. True worship, by contrast, leads us to express His love to our fellow men. Above all, God desires a relationship with His human children, a friendship that can be obtained only through study of His Word, prayer, and meditation. By beholding Him, we are changed into His likeness. His peace in our hearts is the best remedy for the stress of life.

Those who overcome are beautifully described as those who patiently endure the discipline of living godly lives. They keep the commandments of God, not from a feeling of necessity but because they love Him. They are fully aware of their personal weakness, but by God's help, they are strong. They seek to glorify God in their lives, realizing this can only happen as Christ in them becomes their life and hope.

The three angels' messages entail more than physical health, but it seems evident in studying them that God is calling His people to higher living. Unless we surrender our everyday lives to Him—our eating, dressing, resting, exercise, and other habits—we are not truly ready for His Spirit to fill us. What we do moment by moment has little meaning in itself, but it may have immense importance as a measure of our willingness to give God full control.

God seeks to bring mankind back to the perfection in which they were created.[35] He wishes us to "know what are the riches of the glory of this mystery among the Gentiles: which is Christ in you, the hope of glory . . . [presenting] every man perfect in Christ Jesus."[36] The best understanding of "perfection" is to view it as Christian maturity, growing up into Christ.[37] This high standard of living is achievable by "faith in Christ," allowing Him to live His life in us.[38] He is knocking at the door of our hearts and minds, waiting for us to let Him in to even the daily parts of our lives.[39] He will never force Himself, but He is patiently knocking today. Will we let Him in?

Creation "eagerly waits for the revealing of the sons of God."[40] The curtain is rising. We are the final actors in the last scene of earth's history. God, our Director, designs that we be a "spectacle to the world, both to angels and to men."[41]

We are not the stars of this show. God and His love are the glory of this presentation; however, we are important players. Satan has declared that it is impossible to please God, and certainly those who live fleshly lives cannot please Him.[42] But Enoch and other saints through the ages have shown us how to please Him. God now, in these last days, will have a whole generation on the world stage. That's us. Our time has come. Thank God for the direction we have!

> Now may the God of peace Himself sanctify you completely; and may your whole spirit, soul, and body be preserved blameless at the coming of our Lord Jesus Christ. He who calls you is faithful, who also will do it.[43]

Our Director has shown us the script—in His life, His Word, the study of nature and the human body, and through the latter-day prophet, Ellen G. White. Not only that, but He is prepared to coach us intimately, to live our act for us. What more could He do to help us?

The script states that

> the grace of God that brings salvation has appeared to all men, teaching us that, denying ungodliness and worldly lusts, we should live soberly, righteously, and godly in the present age, looking for the blessed hope and glorious appearing of our great God and Savior Jesus Christ, who gave Himself for us, that He might redeem us from every lawless deed and purify for Himself His own special people, zealous for good works.[44]

We are "His own special people"—His children by adoption.

> Behold what manner of love the Father has bestowed on us, that we should be called *children of God!* . . . It has not yet been revealed what we shall be, but we know that when He is revealed, we shall be like Him, for we shall see Him as He is. And everyone who has this hope in Him purifies himself, just as He is pure.[45]

How does one "purify himself"? By beholding and studying the glory of the Lord and allowing the Holy Spirit to transform. "But we all, with unveiled face, beholding as in a mirror the glory of the Lord, are being transformed into the same image from glory to glory, just as by the Spirit of the Lord."[46]

Our Prayer

Thank you, Jesus. You have shown us how to be transformed and live pure lives consecrated to You. It's our turn on the stage in this last drama, and the spotlight is turned on us. Our prayer is that You, by Your Spirit, might be clearly seen in that spotlight. Amen.

---

[1] John 14:6, 7.
[2] John 14:23.
[3] Colossians 1:27, 28.
[4] Acts 26:18.
[5] Galatians 2:20.
[6] Philippians 3:9.
[7] Romans 10:13; Joel 2:32.
[8] Acts 4:12.
[9] Romans 14:23.
[10] 1 Thessalonians 1:3.
[11] John 6:28, 29.
[12] 1 John 3:23.
[13] James 2:17, 18, and 22.
[14] Philippians 2:12, 13.
[15] Psalms 37:3, 6.
[16] 1 Thessalonians 5:23, 24.
[17] Philippians 3:20, 21.
[18] 1 John 3:2, 3.
[19] Philippians 4:13.
[20] Ephesians 3:20, 21.
[21] Romans 12:1.
[22] 1 Corinthians 3:17.
[23] 1 Corinthians 6:20.
[24] Psalm 103:2-5, 13-19.
[25] Isaiah 38:21.
[26] Isaiah 30:21.
[27] James 1:17.
[28] Romans 8:28.
[29] Acts 3:21.
[30] Psalm 51:12, 13.
[31] 1 Peter 4:11.
[32] John 10:10.
[33] Ephesians 3:20, 21.
[34] Ellen G. White, *The Ministry of Healing* (Pacific Press Publishing, 1909) 159, 160.
[35] Ellen G. White, *Education* (Pacific Press Publishing, 1903) 15, 16.
[36] Colossians 1:27, 28.
[37] Ephesians 4:13-15.

[38] Galatians 2:20.
[39] Revelation 3:20.
[40] Romans 8:19.
[41] 1 Corinthians 4:9.
[42] Romans 8:8.
[43] 1 Thessalonians 5:23, 24.
[44] Titus 2:11-14.
[45] 1 John 3:1-3.
[46] 2 Corinthians 3:18.

GLOSSARY

Activated charcoal is produced by the controlled burning of wood which is then subjected to the action of an oxidizing gas such as steam or air at elevated temperatures. Activation enhances the adsorptive power of charcoal—its ability to attract and hold particles to it.

Aerobics refers to a variety of exercises that stimulate heart and lung activity for a time period sufficiently long to produce beneficial changes in the body; this increases the amount of oxygen that the body can process in a given time; concept popularized by Dr. Kenneth H. Cooper.

***Agape* love** is the pure, selfless love of God as described in 1 Corinthians 13; contrasts with *phileo* love, which is based on feelings and emotions, and *eros* love, which refers to sexual passion.

AIDS is acquired immune deficiency syndrome, caused by the human immunodeficiency virus (HIV). It is an almost 100 percent fatal disease acquired by sexual contact or from contaminated body fluids; immune defenses completely break down and death is usually by an opportunistic infection.

Antioxidant is a substance that prevents oxidation—combination with oxygen; oxidation can produce "wild" oxygen molecules (free radicals), which can be harmful; antioxidants protect against harmful oxidized substances.

Anxiety, "free-floating" is a constant state of apprehension, uneasiness, or fear that is often poorly recognized by the anxious person.

Atherosclerosis is disease of blood vessels marked by fatty deposits in the inner layer of arterial walls—atheroma; it can increase, when blood cholesterol remains high, to the point of obstruction of the blood vessel.

Behavior modification refers to the recognition that poor behavior often causes or accentuates disease processes; especially refers to the science of helping people change their poor or bad behaviors.

Beta carotene is the pigment in dark green and yellow vegetables and fruits that the body can convert into vitamin A; a potent antioxidant that can protect against "free radicals," which can cause cancer and other destruction in the body.

Caffeine beverages are liquids that contain caffeine; include tea, coffee, and a vast array of "cola" and other soda pop drinks.

Catecholamines are compounds which have a sympathetic nervous system stimulating effect; include epinephrine (adrenaline) and norepinephrine (noradrenaline).

Character refers to personally developed habits of thought; good character building is the work of a lifetime—a constant struggle to overcome self and impulse; the only thing, with the help of God's Spirit, that we develop on earth and take to heaven.

Cholesterol is a fatty substance found only in animal products; it is produced in the body as a base for hormones and other necessary metabolites; when in excess in the blood, it deposits in blood vessel walls or as kidney or gallstones; is found in many different forms.

Chromosomes are threadlike structures in a cell nucleus; composed primarily of genes which are made of the genetic material, DNA; are in pairs in all cells except the ovum and sperm cells.

Circadian rhythm is the 24-hour sleep/wake cycle and all the biological changes that occur daily.

CNS is the central nervous system; brain and spinal cord; voluntary nervous system.

Complex carbohydrates are the food source preferred by the body and its favorite source of energy; include the starches in grains, legumes, vegetables, and some fruits, in contrast to the simple carbohydrates (the sugars).

Coping refers to the successful struggle against, for instance, stress.

Curds are prepared from milk by placing it in a container and shaking it until it clabbers. Spoken of in the Bible as a symbol of abundance (along with honey).

Dependence is relying on others for social or psychologic support; also refers to chemical addiction where the body adapts to a chemical to the point it is required to make the person function "normally."

Depression is emotional dejection; a morbid sadness, melancholy, or lack of hope frequently accompanied by loss of interest in surroundings and a lack of energy.

Diet is one's food intake; bodily nourishment; often relates to rules for eating.

Differentiation is a genetic term to describe the process of cells changing from a single cell (at conception) to become all the different specialized cells that make up a human body.

Discipline is the training of the mind and character; refers to control, order, obedience to rules.

Distillation is the process of evaporation and condensation; extracting the essence of something.

DNA is deoxyribonucleic acid, the nuclear molecule which directs and controls all activity in the cell; the basis for heredity; contains the "code of life."

Efficiency refers to the degree of effectiveness; doing the most possible with the least effort or energy.

Emotion is a strong feeling such as joy, fear, or anger.

Endorphins are hormone substances produced in the brain which are capable of producing euphoria (good feelings) and relieving pain.

Enzymes are protein molecules which promote or accelerate chemical changes; each enzyme is a catalyst of only one activity but does not become a part of that which is produced.

Euphoria is a feeling of well-being.

Evaluate means to determine or assess the value or success of something.

Evolution is the continued, gradual change from one form or state to another; a belief in the spontaneous and random development of life and its forms over long time spans.

Exercise refers to the use of the muscles of the body in an effort to increase their power or efficiency; physical exertion for health improvement; voluntary muscle activity.

Extrinsic refers to something originating externally (outside).

Feeling is the sense of touch; an emotion or a conscious or unconscious personal interpretation of a life experience; an intuitive belief.

Fiber, dietary is found only in plants—fruits, vegetables, whole grains, and legumes; is found in two forms: insoluble (crude) fiber and water soluble fiber such as gums and pectin.

Fibrosis is fibrous (scar) tissue formation; an abnormal degenerative process.

Fitness is a state of well-being that enables one to perform daily work without undue fatigue.

Free radicals are unstable (wild) oxygen molecules that have an electron structure which causes them to be attracted to other oxygen-containing substances and can cause oxidation or serious damage to structures in the body such as DNA, blood vessel walls, etc.

Genes are the hereditary units which occupy fixed positions in chromosomes; they manage the formation of cellular protein.

Habit is a constant tendency; a pattern or action which becomes automatic after frequent repetition; a chemical addiction.

HDL cholesterol is the high-density lipoproten portion of cholesterol; it is "good" cholesterol in that it tends to collect the lipid and transport it to the liver, where it is broken down and excreted. Ideally should be in the blood at a level above 45 mg/dl of blood. It is increased best by long, slow, distance exercise, losing weight, and stopping smoking.

Healing is the process of returning to normal; improved health.

Health reform has in the past been a term suggesting need for change or improvement in providing medical care; the term is currently used in the U.S. to identify the need to hold down or decrease the high costs of health care.

Hectare is the metric measure of land; 10,000 sq. meters or 2.471 acres.

Herbs are plants used as food, seasoning, or medicine. Many plant substances are toxic and need to be taken cautiously as medicine; dosage is usually not standardized and purity is often questionable.

Homeostasis is a state of equilibrium (balance) within the body; self-regulated maintenance of body processes or substances.

Hormone is a chemical substance secreted by a gland cell which regulates specific body cells by slowing or speeding target cell activity.

Hostility is an antagonistic attitude toward another person.

Hydrotherapy is the therapeutic application of hot or cold water in various forms—directly, in cloths, vapor, etc.

Hypertonic fatigue is "nervous" fatigue that manifests itself in tensed muscles; insomnia (inability to sleep) often occurs with this type of tiredness.

Hypoglycemia is the body condition brought on by low blood sugar (below 80 mg/dl in the blood).

Hypotonic fatigue is weariness brought on by muscular work or exercise; muscles are relaxed and sleep comes easily.

Illicit drugs are illegal drugs.

Immune system includes all the organs or cells in the body which, combined together, protect against infectious organisms or harmful substances.

Interstitial refers to gaps or spaces between cells; usually filled by serous fluid.

Intrinsic refers to belonging or situated entirely within a body or part.

Isolation is the experience of being separated from a group; set apart by oneself; having no meaningful contacts with others.

Kcal is a kilocalorie (large calorie); a measure of the energy-producing value of food according to the amount of heat it produces when oxidized within the body; the amount of heat required to raise the temperature of one kilogram of water one degree centigrade.

LDL Cholesterol is low-density lipoprotein cholesterol; the "bad" cholesterol that tends to collect in the blood vessel walls in atheromatous plaques. It is associated with high fat and cholesterol food intake. Should be below 120 mg/dl in the blood.

Legumes are all the beans, peas and lentils; edible seeds enclosed in pods, used in both dry and fresh states; rich in protein.

Longevity refers to actual or expected life span in years.

Medical missionary work is the activity of unselfish love and compassion shown toward those in need; it is the gospel in practice; its object is to point sin-sick people to their Saviour; it does not necessarily include medical care and can be as simple as rejoicing with them that rejoice and weeping with them that weep—being kindly affectioned one to another. Romans 12.

Metabolism refers to the chemical and physical processes which take place in the body that are necessary for life; especially those processes involving use of food and oxygen (energy breakdown and production).

Miracle is an unexpected event that cannot be explained by natural law; a supernatural intervention in human affairs

Molecule is the smallest unit of distinct chemical substances; made up of two or more atoms.

Natural law governs the normal functioning of biologic organisms; it is the divine plan which regulates body functions; God's physical law—e.g. the laws of health.

Natural remedies are natural substances used to treat sickness; often these are folk medicine used at home; should always cooperate with normal physiologic function—obey nature's laws.

NREM sleep is "non-rapid eye movement" deep sleep, usually early in the night, when the body is physically recovering from fatigue; alternates with REM sleep; is slow-wave sleep.

Nucleolus a small, spherical organelle located in the cell nucleus; it is an active center for protein and RNA synthesis.

Nucleus is the central part of the cell which contains the chromosomes; controls metabolism, growth, and reproduction.

Nutrients are components of foods which are essential to life; **essential nutrients** usually refers to nutrients which cannot be manufactured by the body—must come from foods; **basic nutrients** refers to the minimum number and type of food components required by the body for life.

Nutrition is the process of taking food and utilizing it in the body; includes digestion, absorption, metabolism and excretion.

Optimum is the most favorable or best quality available.

Oxidation is the combining of a substance with oxygen; a chemical reaction in which an electron is transferred from one molecule to another.

Phagocytic activity refers to cells ingesting bacteria, foreign particles, or other cells.

Photoreceptors are specialized cells, for instance in the retina, which chemically register light and then stimulate nerve transmission into the brain, thus enabling sight.

Physiology is the science of the normal function and activity of living organisms.

Phytochemicals are plant chemicals which are not nutrients but do affect health by working against cancer cells and other diseases; they are newly discovered and were not really recognized until the 1990s; identifying active plant chemicals which promote health is a new era in nutrition.

Potable water is pure drinking water.

Precipitating cause is the activity which brings about or makes evident a disease or malfunction in the body.

Precursor is anything that in the course of a process precedes or is a forerunner of a later stage; an inactive substance that is converted to an active substance such as a hormone or enzyme.

Psychoactive is something that speeds or slows down mental activity.

Psychosis is severe mental illness marked by loss of contact with reality; can include childish behavior, delusions, or hallucinations.

Psychotoxic refers to chemical poisoning of the mind.

Psychotropic drugs (chemicals) are chemicals which speed up or slow down the activity of the mind or actually poison it; altered brain function almost always disturbs the higher brain functions of judgment, perception, discrimination, will-power, etc.

Reaction effect is an effect that is opposite to that which originated the reaction; e.g. the reaction of the body to cold can be the production of heat in the body.

Recreation refers to activities that bring about renewal, refreshment, or regeneration of body, mind, and spirit.

Reflex is an involuntary and immediate response to a stimulus; it is mediated through the nervous system and may affect a part at some distant from the site of the stimulus.

REM sleep is "rapid eye movement" sleep when the eyes can be observed to be moving rapidly back and forth; alternates with NREM sleep; it is the time when dreams occur and appears to be used by the mind to consolidate memory and organize and rejuvenate the nervous system.

Resistance is any force that opposes and/or retards motion; a psychologic defense mechanism in which a person unconsciously represses recall of certain events or experiences.

Restraint is to forcibly control or hinder.

Reverse osmosis is the movement by external pressure of a solution through a semi-permeable membrane from an area of lesser density to one of a higher density or concentration.

RHR is resting heart rate; ideally obtained while in bed just after awakening.

Risk refers to the potential of disease or injury; risk factors are the conditions that predispose persons to disease or injury.

RNA is ribonucleic acid; relays messages from the DNA to the ribosomes and other cell structures.

Sanctification is to make holy, consecrate, set apart, separate from common use; it denotes a process of character development—learning to live a holy, perfect life; it is the work of a lifetime and can be successful only by the power and grace of God.

Sidestream smoke refers to the unfiltered smoke that passes directly from the burning tobacco; has a higher concentration of some harmful compounds than does "mainstream" smoke; secondhand smoke has been proven to cause cancer and other disease in the nonsmokers who breathe it.

Social support refers to the assistance others can provide persons in times of crisis or special need; ideally all churches should consider themselves as compassionate, nonjudgmental social support units for sinners who feel their need.

Stressor is the stimulus, usually adverse, which tends to disturb the homeostasis or balance of a person; the agent or condition which produces stress.

Sunscreens are preparations designed to be put on skin to block the cancer-producing UV rays of the sun; the higher the number on the sunscreen preparation, the greater its blocking effect; sunscreens with an index number of 15 or higher are most recommended..

SWS is slow-wave sleep; it is the same as NREM sleep; assists the recovery from physical fatigue.

Triglycerides are dietary fats found in the blood; they are the major storage form of fat found in the adipose (fat) tissues; in large amounts cause the blood to be sluggish.

Ultrafiltration is passage through a filter which is capable of removing all but the very smallest particles; refers to forcing water through a membrane or barrier which removes at least 99 percent of all solid particles.

UV light is the range of invisible light from the visible violet portion of light out to the low-frequency x-ray portion of the electromagnetic spectrum; the most harmful portion of sunlight; it is associated with cataracts and skin cancer, especially melanomas.

Vaccination is injection or ingestion of a substance which stimulates the body's immune system to produce active immunity against the substance; the substance is usually a solution containing dead or live attenuated viruses or bacteria.

Values are the personal estimates or worth placed on objects or experiences.

Vegetarians are persons who choose to eat only plant products and refuse to eat any animal products; ovo-lacto vegetarians eat no meat, fish, or fowl but do eat milk products and eggs.

Virus is a very small infectious organism capable of only living in living cells; many are RNA or DNA particles which enter cells and disrupt normal DNA or RNA function, producing uncontrolled growth (tumors).

Viscosity refers to the resistance of a liquid to flow; a viscous substance may be sticky or glutinous and have a high resistance to flowing.